KETOGENIC DIET:

The Ketogenic Diet Cookbook with 100 + unique recipes to Heal your Body & Lose Weight

TABLE OF CONTENTS

INTRODUCTION

You've tried every diet out there, with minimal long-term results or possibly none at all! Perhaps you love your low-carb or Paleo diet, but is it enough to kick your metabolism into full gear and burn that extra weight in order to achieve a healthier lifestyle? By eating great sources of good fats, moderate protein, and just a bit of carbohydrates, your body will feel less hungry, less cravings and ultimately feel better.

Not only that, your body will begin to burn off stored fat instead of the glucose and carbohydrates that usually bring down your system and leaves you feeling exhausted.

Over the past several decades, we've been provided with dietary advice that has been repeatedly proven inaccurate. Physicians and nutritionists know that various studies starting from the 1950s have been severely manipulated as many of these studies received funding the companies that produce foods and additives that are not exactly good for us.

These studies focus on the foundation of the food pyramid that has been taught in school since the late 1950s and led us to believe is a "balanced diet".

The ketogenic diet was originally developed by Dr. Russell Wilder at the Mayo Clinic in 1924. It was proven to be very effective in treating epilepsy in children that did not respond to medication. Despite these studies showing just how effective the diet was, it fell out of favor after the discovery of the new anti-seizure medications in the late 1940s.

Here, you will discover the science behind the ketogenic diet and learn how to make this diet work for YOU. Indulge in recipes that are specifically created to for ketogenic, high-fat, low-carb, grain-free, gluten-free, ancestral, primal and Paleo diets.

The Ketogenic Diet Cookbook contains over 100 recipes along with how to use the ketogenic diet as a better way of life. Not only are the recipes simple and easy to prepare, they are also specifically designed to support ketosis in your body and allow you to heal from the inside. Unlike any other ketogenic diet cook, we've written a complete guide with important Keto facts and flavourful healthy recipes to kick-start your ketogenic lifestyle.

Discover how to gain the benefits of the ketogenic diet, with:

- Over 100 delicious, easy-to-follow recipes

- Complete overview explaining the ins and outs of the ketogenic diet

- Keto-friendly foods to help you make your own plan

Are you ready to make a better change? Let's get started!

CHAPTER 1. WHAT IS THE KETOGENIC DIET?

My Story

My story began a couple years ago after a series of health scares that forced me to take a better look at my horrible diet and unhealthy habits. I started my weight loss journey in 2014 in hopes of improving my health and overall well-being.

My blood pressure was elevated, and I started having issues with sudden plain in my feet and blurred vision. What truly terrified me was that I started having the same symptoms my father had before he was diagnosed with Diabetes. So I started paying more attention to the foods I ate, slowly changing my diet.

In the beginning, I cut out the obvious unhealthy junk foods and started eating REAL food. I ditched the canned and instant meals and starting cooking my own with fresh vegetables and lean meats instead. While my diet was better and I removed most of the harmful foods, I still gave into my cravings and ate chocolate or chips occasional throughout the week.

Within six months, I noticed a big change and wanted to learn more about eating healthy and which foods can make a difference in your health. I soon found out that "healthy eating" is the exact opposite of what mainstream medicine and the federal government were saying.

I then discovered that the whole-grain, low-fat, high-carb diet that was highly encouraged by the USDA was actually making people sick, not making them live longer and better. I also learned that saturated fat and cholesterol was not the evil culprit that causes heart disease and damage to our health.

While I was making changes to my new healthy habits, I soon realized that the less sugar and bread I ate, the better I felt. After expressing my enthusiasm to a friend, it was when she mentioned the ketogenic diet. Immediately, I started doing research and tried it. After the first month on the ketogenic diet, I stuck to 20 carbohydrates a day, and then worked my way up to about 30 then 50 carbohydrates a day. I lost 20 pounds and felt better than ever, even without any exercise.

Within a week or two, the weight loss stopped as I stuck to an average 50 carbs per day. I started losing motivation and questioning how effective the keto diet really was. Following the plan completely, I even dropped my calorie intake to 1300 a day in hopes of losing more weight. This became very discouraging when I'd look 5 pounds and gain 2 more back.

However, I noticed a significantly large improve to my health while losing some weight. So I stuck with it. At some point I realized that whole-grain products made me feel terrible, so I decided to cut out grains from my diet. While I didn't lose any weight with this diet change, I did notice my energy levels were increases, my skin looked amazing and I felt overall super healthy.

During my struggles to be healthy, eat better and lose weight, I became convinced that a normal weight and great health that the best results anyone could ask for.

That's my story. I hope this helps you in your own personal journey. If you are struggling with health or weight issues, please know that you can and WILL succeed, if you stick to this plan and make the necessary changes. It may seem quite difficult at first but you will soon adapt to a new way of living, and eating will become easier.

What is a Ketogenic Diet?

The ketogenic diet is a low-carbohydrate, moderate-protein, high-fat diet that was originally used to help treat epilepsy in children who did not respond to medicine.

This diet forces the body to burn fat instead of carbohydrates for energy. The body converts the carbohydrates into glucose which is then used as energy throughout the body. Unfortunately, taking in more carbohydrates than you need will cause the excess glucose to be converted into stored fat rather than be eliminated. However, restricting carbohydrates will cause the liver to convert fat into ketone bodies and fatty acids. Once the ketones in the blood outnumber the glucose molecules, the cells will begin using ketose as a source of energy.

How does a Ketogenic Diet Work?

The ketogenic diet alters the body's metabolism from using glucose to ketones as energy. While this diet does not guarantee fast weight loss like other traditional diets, it is however an effective tool to help you reach your goals of living a healthy lifestyle and eating better.

With this diet you will eat both satisfying and nutritious foods that will make you less hunger and have fewer cravings. According to medical studies, good fats cause satiation while fruits and vegetables do not. Fats and protein are the most satisfying of the 3 macronutrients that you will learn about in this eBook.

Eating good sources of fats will actually help your body burn fat that is already stored to help you lose weight easier as carbohydrates signal the body to produce insulin to move glucose molecules into the cells for energy.

However, if one has been overweight for a long period of time, they will be more at risk of experiences some form of insulin-resistance, even without being diagnosed as a diabetic. Meaning you will also experience high and low blood sugar levels as well as cravings.

With the ketogenic diet, you will be able to achieve a successful weight loss due to the metabolic advantage of the low-carb diet. As your liver works to break down fats, more ketones will be excreted through urination.

Can the Ketogenic Diet be Dangerous?

You may have heard that the ketogenic diet can be dangerous to your health. However, these "dangers" are myths passed on by those with a limited understand of just how low-carb diets work.

One of the main sources of criticism is that this is a high-fat diet that may cause you to develop a risk of heart-related problems. The idea that fat is what makes you fat has been constantly drilled into the brains of Americans over the past 30 years. While it is difficult to unlearn lies that you've been taught all of your life, the reality is that a high-carb diet can increase your blood sugar and insulin levels.

Sugar and insulin can cause inflammation while the allowed fats in the ketogenic diet are healthy saturated fats. This saturated fats and high levels of sugar is combined in the standard American diet, it becomes the "cause" of heart disease.

Another criticism of the Ketogenic diet is that high amounts of cholesterol and saturated fats cause heart disease, another lie that has been embedded to our brains for decades. A study from John Hopkins Medical School states that the ketogenic diet is proven to be healthier due to the high amounts of saturated fat intake.

While low carbohydrate intakes decrease triglyceride levels, high intakes of saturated fat increase HDL – *the good cholesterol.* The closer your HDL and triglyceride levels are to 1, the healthier your heart is. It is said that heart disease is caused by high amounts of carbohydrates on a daily basis.

There are also saying that people don't do well in ketosis, which isn't entirely true. As we will discuss this later in the book, be sure to consult with your physician or nutritionist before starting the ketogenic diet if you have pre-existing medical conditions.

Keep in mind that it has been discovered that our caveman ancestors survived a constant state of ketosis due to difficult in gathering grains in large amounts and were not as processed as carbohydrates are today.

Another cause of criticism is the danger of falling into ketoacidosis during the ketogenic diet. Ketoacidosis is a life-threatening condition that occurs when there is an abnormally high level of ketones in the blood caused by an unregulated biochemical reaction. Although ketosis is not enough to put you at risk of developing this condition

Ketoacidosis generally occurs in people diagnosed with Type 1 diabetes. Nutritional ketosis is a regulated process that allows insulin to remain in the blood in order to counteract the ketones which will prevent a healthy individual from develop ketoacidosis.

The only ways for someone to develop ketoacidosis while following the ketogenic diet are:

- Going under starvation mode for several months – which should not occur with a formulated meal plan.

- Perform long periods of extremely high-intensity exercise.

- Chronic alcoholics who indulge in binges in extreme measures.

As you can see, following a nutritional ketosis is not dangerous when properly planned. This diet is a natural metabolic process that is safe for anyone who is not a diabetic who lacks insulin or severe alcoholics.

CHAPTER 2. WHAT I SHOULD KNOW BEFORE STARTING THE KETOGENIC DIET

As with every diet, there are a few measures that you should consider and know before starting the ketogenic diet. First, you must be patient with yourself. There may be side effects as your metabolism changes. You may also experience rapid weight-loss followed by a plateau once your diet is regulated. Just don't be discouraged as it is just your body adjusting to the new amount of energy being provided.

Second, be sure to discuss your plans with your physician to be sure that this diet is for you. Your health is important and you don't want to endanger it in the process of trying to actually improve it. Most medical doctors are not specialized in nutrition and may not understand the difference between ketoacidosis and nutritional ketosis. While ketoacidosis is extremely life-threatening, it is extremely rare that only occurs in people who are unable to produce insulin and not diagnosed with Type 1 diabetes.

Most medical professionals usually do not offer advice that is not generally accepted. If that is the case with your doctor, don't be surprised if they can't find a reason for your weight loss and overall health improvement.

Last, understand the side effects that you may experience and how you can ease these symptoms.

What are the Early Stages of Ketosis?

During the early stages of ketosis, your body will begin to adapt to the presence of ketones in the blood stream with some unpleasant symptoms. As your body balances itself out, the symptoms will decrease.

As with any diet, changing your daily eating habits to the ketogenic lifestyle is not easy. However, once you have adapted to this newfound lifestyle, you will discover how much healthier and better you feel.

Understand that these side effects are temporary and will last for only a few days up to a month. Learning to understand your body's physical reactions will help you find a way to minimize them and save you from the misery caused by carbohydrate withdrawal.

Let's start with the bad news before we continue on to the amazing benefits of following the ketogenic diet.

Possible Side Effects

- Frequent urination
- Dizziness and Fatigue
- Headache and Muscle Cramps
- Hypoglycemia
- Dry Mouth
- Constipation
- Sugar Cravings
- Diarrhea

- Sleep Changes
- Kidney Stones
- Metallic taste in the mouth
- Low T3 Thyroid Hormone levels
- Heart Palpitations
- Hair Loss
- Cold hands and feet

Dealing with the Side Effects

As Ketosis is common on a low-carb diet, the side effects aren't always pleasant. If you find yourself struggling through this period, here are some ways to help ease symptoms:

★ **Have Regular Snacks**

Have a protein-rich snack like chicken to help ease symptoms and headaches.

★ **Drink Plenty of Water**

Drinking enough water will keep your body hydrated and freshen your breath.

★ **Try a Protein Shake**

Protein shakes contained with amino acid supplements will help reduce symptoms of ketosis and ease the transition.

★ **Take Vitamins and Minerals**

Due to the lack of fruits and vegetables, it is vital to take a good-quality supplement to help keep your body in balance.

Benefits of the Ketogenic Diet

As your body begins to adapt to ketones, your symptoms will start to slowly change or disappear altogether. While your urine may still show present ketones, it will probably be in low concentrations.

You will know you've adapted to ketones by the following symptoms:

- Less Hunger Pangs
- Lower Blood Pressure
- Lower Levels of Cholesterol
- Lower Blood Sugar and Insulin Levels
- Increased Levels of Energy
- Less Joint Pain and Stiffness
- Reduced Fogginess; Clear thinking
- Stabilized Sleeping patterns
- Normalized urination
- Weight Loss
- Gastric Symptoms Relief
- Improvement in Oral Health
- Increased Dopamine and Serotonin Levels

It is impossible however for low-carb dieters to never reach ketosis. This could be due to exercise using up the excess ketones or diluted urine from drinking plenty of water. But this doesn't mean you are not burning fat.

Who should not follow a Ketogenic Diet?

While the ketogenic diet has been proven safe for almost everyone, there are still certain people with conditions that **should not** follow this diet and lifestyle.

Metabolic Conditions

- Type 1 Diabetes
- Primary Carnitine Deficiency
- Carnitine palmitoyltransferase (CPT) Type 1 or 2 deficiency
- Carnitine translocase deficiency
- Defects of Beta-oxidation
- Impaired liver function
- Malnutrition
- Gastric bypass surgery
- Abdominal tumors
- Impaired gastric motility (this can be due to cancer treatment and medications)
- Kidney failure
- If you are pregnant or breastfeeding
- Porphyria
- Pancreatitis
- Gall Bladder disease

How Does a Ketogenic Diet Compare to Other Diets?

You may have tried at least one – *or many* of the popular diets and experiences a few months-worth of easy weight loss. But once that fad diet became boring, this also leads to completely ruining your dieting efforts. Am I right?

Let's compare how a traditional diet and the ketogenic diet can both achieve your weight loss goals.

Traditional Diet:

- Allows moderate protein intake
- Increase high fruit and vegetable intake
- Restricts fat intake
- Restricts caloric intake

- Follows the Dietary Food Pyramid Guideline
- Not easily adjustable to reduce hunger
- Doesn't relieve cravings

Ketogenic Diet:

- Allows moderate protein intake
- Increases "good" fat intake
- Restricts carbohydrate intake
- Doesn't force caloric restriction
- Allows adjustment to reduce hunger
- Alleviates cravings

As you may notice, the ketogenic diet is the total opposite of any popular, trending traditional diet that you may have already tried. Maybe that's why more and more people are becoming success stories!

CHAPTER 3: HOW TO START THE KETOGENIC DIET

Counting Macros vs. Calories

If you've been trying to learn more about the ketogenic, you've probably already heard about "macros" macronutrients. In this section, we are going to discuss whether you should be counting macros or calories and the differences between them.

If you learn the how to calculate the proper proportions of macros, then the ketogenic diet will become much easier to follow rather than restricting calories that would most likely cause you to fail.

As traditional diets generally consider the calories you consume rather than *what* you eat, this method is often a set up for failure. While portion control can work for a few months, this will lead to a serious bring and even cause you to give up on the diet altogether. Your self-control will eventually break down unless you are eating the right foods.

Concentrating on counting macronutrients will help you eat more of the right foods. This will also help you to stay motivated and stick to your diet.

What are Macronutrients?

Macros, or macronutrients that the foods that provide energy for your cells. Your macros are the 3 important nutrients, which includes carbohydrates, fats and proteins. Each macronutrient provides energy when they are broken as down and comes in the form of calories.

Every single gram of proteins and carbohydrates will break down during digestion and provide 4 solid calories. However, Fats provide 9 calories per gram that is broken down by our digestive system.

Carbohydrates

Technically, your body CAN survive without carbohydrates but you will still have to find the amount of glucose than your brain needs from protein. When your body breaks down protein into glucose, it actually uses more energy than it provides – making carbohydrates a good thing *in small amounts,* of course.

Protein

Protein is linked to building muscle tissue, although it is also the main component in all tissues and organs of your body, hair, and enzymes. It is made up of amino acids that are required for proper functioning, that our bodies can make for ourselves. However, there are nine essential amino acids that you must get from food as they are mainly found in meats.

Fats

Fats have a bad reputation because they are rich in calories. However, fats are very important in order to normalize bodily functions. Fats surround each nerve to protect tissues, conduct impulse, make up the backbone of our hormones, and make our hair and skin strong and healthy.

While there are many types of fats in our diets like saturated, polyunsaturated, monounsaturated, trans-fat and more – the ones you should eat are Omega-3 and Omega-6 fatty acids. Just be careful of how much you eat as eating too much omega-6 will cause an increase in inflammation in your muscles and joints.

Do Calories Count on the Ketogenic Diet?

While counting macros is an important factor in the ketogenic diet, counting calories will also help too. Consider this another tool in your diet to simply reduce calorie intake. Just be sure to remember that you don't necessarily need to eat that many calories.

Example: a 40 year old women weights 285 lbs. and is 5'7, living a sedentary lifestyle. To maintain her weight, she would need about 2,300 calories a day. If they reduced that amount to 1,800, she would lose about 1 pound a week. However, with the right food combination, she may never reach up to 1800 calories a day on the ketogenic diet. This will result to an increase in weight loss.

The fats and protein you eat will offer enough satiation to keep you from feeling hungry. While vegetables will provide you with enough fiber to feel full. This will increase your metabolic rate and cause you to burn more calories than you would on a traditional diet.

Muscle Building and Weight Loss

Most individuals who start following the ketogenic lifestyle are not always fit. However, this doesn't mean your body can't get to that point once you've reached your ideal weight and desired level of health.

Once your body becomes fully adapted to this diet and you have lost weight, you will begin to feel more energy and adjust your menus to accommodate building muscle mass and strength.

As you reach the point of feeling like muscle building and toning is right for you, you will then be able to alter the diet to what is called "cyclical" or "targeted." Both versions will allow you to consume more carbohydrates so that you can gain enough glucose to feed your muscles without coming out of ketosis.

The cyclical ketogenic diet will allow you to add more carbohydrates during exercise times in order to allow you to perform a high-intensity workout without falling out of ketosis. This will be very beneficial as you will have the necessary glucose to work your muscles.

Keep in mind that the cyclical ketogenic diet is more realistic for advanced bodybuilders and athletic trainers as it is used to build maximum muscle. This will not work for beginners as it can take up to 3 weeks for your body to go into ketosis.

This stage of the ketogenic diet will have you follow the standard ketogenic diet for 5-6 days with 1-2 days of having a high-carb intake. If you choose to go on this diet, then you must complete deplete your body's amount of glycogen during your training session.

Is it possible to NOT lose weight on the Ketogenic Diet?

In the case where you are not losing weight and finding it difficult to get into the state of ketosis or you've been experiencing times of stress that is making it hard for you to keep your lifestyle. This can be due to stress from the holidays, eating out more often, or stopping in general.

Is it possible to not lose weight? **Yes.** It is quite possible for you to experience a lack of weight loss while following a ketogenic diet. However, there are several reasons that can be dealt with by making certain adjustments to your diet and lifestyle.

- Eating too many Carbohydrates

- Eating the Wrong Amounts of Protein

- Cheating on Carbs

- Eating too much Fat

- Consuming too many Artificial Sweeteners

- Excessive Amounts of Nuts and Dairy

- Close to your Target Weight

- Overstressed

- Circadian Rhythms might be disrupted

- Excessive Exercise

- Might have an Adrenal or Thyroid Issue

- Lack of Leptin Production

- Lack of Water and Electrolytes

What to Do If I Plateau?

As with any kind of diet, plateauing is not unexpected when it comes to the ketogenic diet. When you start to lose weight, your metabolism will also decline. This will cause you to burn fewer calories than you did at your heavier weight.

The slower your metabolism becomes, the harder it will become for you to lose weight while eating the same amount of calories. Once you begin to burn the same amount of calories you eat, then you will reach a plateau.

However, there are a few ways to break that cycle and continue to lose weight until you start exercising and strength building.

Eat More Sources of Fiber

Add psyllium husk to your food as a thickener as well as your ketogenic bread. Consuming additional fiber will help reduce your food intake while keeping you feeling full longer.

Acknowledge Your Attitude towards Food

Knowing which moods motivate you to eat will help you determine how to overcome those negative tendencies. If you are anxious, nervous or depressed, you might notice that you find comfort through eating, which is called emotional hunger.

Emotional hunger is often overwhelming and makes you crave certain foods. Unfortunately, those cravings are often fatty or sugary foods. While fatty foods on the ketogenic diet aren't necessarily bad for you, the fatty foods you might crave may not be the beneficial fats that are highly encouraged in your keto diet.

If you are prone to emotional hunger, you will often feel regret and shame after which can lead to more emotional eating. While it is difficult to overcome, it is still possible. Remember that emotional eating is caused by unpleasant feelings and is often used as a reward for celebration. Keep in mind that we must stop treating food as a reward, as it is a way of survival.

To get yourself out of the habit of emotional eating, here's what you can do:

- **Identify what triggers you**. Do you feel stressed or uncomfortable? Are you exhausted or bored? Is rewarding yourself with food a childhood habit? Do you feel nervous when you eat out?

- **Learn to distract your emotional eating thoughts**. Do positive activities such as playing with your kids or walking the dog. Call a friend or family member or go dancing. Read a book, explore new places, work on a hobby, or enjoy a cup of tea – anything to get your mind off eating emotionally.

- **Make time for yourself**. No matter how busy your schedule may be, take 30 minutes to exercise, meditate, or have a nap. Spend time with people who enhance your lift in a positive way.

Fasting & Intermitted Exercise

Fasting and high intensity, intermittent exercises can help break a plateau and put you back on the right track with weight loss. Fasting once in a while is good for your body as it will cleanse the built-up toxins and kick-start your metabolism into high gear. Intermittent high intensity exercise can jump start your metabolism by improving your glucose while burning off excess calories. Due to the intensity, any glycol that remains in the muscles will become depleted and help you stay in ketosis. Since glycol requires stored water, you will then have more water weight to lose.

Intermittent High-Intensity Exercise

Also known as interval training, this exercise technique will alternate intense anaerobic exercise with short periods of recovery. This will make you burn more calories in a short amount of time compared to low-intensity training. The theory behind the anaerobic exercise is to cause muscles to feel tired in a short amount of time.

Here are some suggested forms of exercises that can be accomplished within a 10-minute period of high interval intensity exercise.

- Heavyweight lighting
- High-speed burpees

- Sprinting

- Jump Rope

- Kettle Bell Swings

Intermittent Fasting

Just as it may sound, you will fast for 14-36 hours with a strict feeding period. For longer fasting periods, you have the option of splitting your window in two, if needed.

- Fasting for 14 hours, feeding period of 2-3 hours.

- Fasting for 24 hours, feeding period of 4-6 hours.

- Fasting for 36 hours, feeding period of 6-8 hours.

During your fasting, you can eat as much as you want during your feeding period but will not eat anything except water during your fasting period.

Feeding Period

During this time, you can try to reach your macronutrient goal without restriction. It may not be possible to reach your target and that is okay. Be sure to eat all of your protein. Eating less protein that you need will cause you to lose muscle, decrease your metabolic rate and burn less body fat.

Eat as many fats as necessary and save the carbohydrates for last – keeping it less than 20g.

Fasting Period

During your fasting, you will only be allowed to consume water or any zero caloric beverages. Black coffee and tea are also allowed.

While neither the intermittent fasting nor the high-intensity intermittent is good for weight loss, they will be used as tools to break through the stubborn plateau. Once your body has gotten back to losing weight, you will then be able to adjust your caloric and macronutrient intake.

CHAPTER 4: CREATE YOUR MEAL PLAN

In this section, we will go over the fundamentals of the Ketogenic Diet which may appear to be a bit overwhelming. Do not let the "Avoid" list discourage you as I promise there will be plenty of options to keep you from boring diet meals. Along with a list of approved foods, we will also provide a sample meal plan along with over 100 recipes to compliment your ketogenic meal plan.

Do I need Any Particular Gear?

While this is optional, there are a few kitchen equipment that can make it easier for you to observe each ketogenic recipe.

★ **Blender**

A blender will assist you in achieving pureed results for soups and sauces.

★ **Processor**

A meals processor with a grating/shredding blade is helpful in saving time during preparations.

★ **Mandolin**

A mandolin will allow you to slice julienne and ribbon your greens in a short amount of time.

★ **Vegetable Spiralizer**

The veggie spiralizer will come in handy when making "spaghetti."

★ **Juicer**

For recipes that call for juices, this will turn your fruits and vegetables into juice within seconds.

★ **Digital Kitchen Scale**

As measuring cups are not always the same in all locations, the digital kitchen scale will measure your meals by weight.

★ **Steamer**

A steamer will allow you to steam your vegetables without losing the essential vitamins.

★ **Zester**

As most recipes include lemon, lime or orange zest, a zester will definitely come in handy.

★ **Meals Saver**

Using a vacuum sealing unit will allow you to preserve your meals longer and save for later use.

How to Determine Your Numbers

The key to the Ketogenic lifestyle is to keep in mind that you are replacing carbohydrates with high fats and moderate protein. While fats have a limited effect on insulin production and blood sugar levels in your body, protein affects both when you eat more than your body needs.

The recommended daily intake of protein should be 0.36g per pound. However, today's common diet suggests higher amounts that your body actually requires, which means the extra protein that is not broken down will become glucose and stored as fat. The high amount of glucose will boost insulin levels and stall the body's ability to release and burn off excess ketones.

The ketogenic diet works best when you keep track of your carb intake. All ketogenic plans allow a broad range of grams of carbohydrates per day, around 20-60g daily. However, if you are beginning the new lifestyle, be sure to limit your carb intake to less than 20g a day.

The amount of protein you should consume is not based on your current weight but on your goal weight, gender, and physical exercise. Those who follow a moderately active lifestyle will require more protein that those with a sedentary lifestyle.

So how do you determine the gram and percentages of each macronutrient you need for the ketogenic diet? Let me show you how.

Example 1

Stacy is a 30-year-old woman, 5'7", 250 lbs. and works as a receptionist with very limited exercise. Her ideal weight is about 135 lbs.

Protein intake: 135 x 0.36 = 48.6 grams per day

Stacy's intake of protein will be rounded up to 49 grams and be set at 20% protein. This amount will give her the right amount of essential amino acids that her body needs in order to properly function without a raise in insulin and blood glucose levels. Next, she will determine her carbohydrate percentage. Let's say that Stacy chooses 5% as her carb intake.

Carbohydrate: 49 / 4 = 12.25 grams per day

Stacy will round her grams to 12 grams of carbohydrates per day. Avoiding grains, starchy vegetables, and most fruits will give her plenty of vegetables to eat while maintaining her carbohydrate intake. Now Stacy will need to figure out her daily allowed fat consumption. This is easier since the remaining 75% of her diet should consist of healthy fats.

Fats: (49 x 3) + (12 x 3) = 183 grams per day

Thus, making Stacy's ketogenic 75:20:5 intake; 183 g of Fats, 49g of Protein and 12g of carbohydrates.

Example 2

Stacy's doctor is allowing her to try the ketogenic diet while keeping a close watch on her healthy. However, the doctor suggested that Stacy must combine counting calories as well. Stacy and her doctor have agreed that a 1500 calorie diet would allow Stacy to lose weight without starvation as she follows the ketogenic diet.

Fats: 1500 x 0.75 = 1125 calories

125 cal. / 9 calories per gram = 125 grams per day.

Protein: 1500 x 0.20 = 300 calories

300 / 4 = 75 grams per day.

Carbohydrate: 1500 x 0.05 = 75 calories

75 / 4 = 18.75 grams per day.

As this amount is slightly more than the pure percentage calculation, Stacy has the option to reduce this amount if she chooses. Both options will allow Stacy to lose weight and start feeling better as she slims down. The new energy level will give her the opportunity to increase exercise.

If you are going to count calories while you follow this diet, you will need to reduce your caloric intake. Adjust your meal plan by recalculating your grams per day with a new calorie amount.

Foods You Can Eat

Fats

- Avocado Oil
- Almond Oil
- Beef Tallow; grass fed cattle
- Butter; natural preferred
- chicken Fat
- Duck Fat
- Ghee
- Lard; natural preferred
- Macadamia Oil
- Mayonnaise, no-carb
- Olive Oil
- Sesame Oil
- Flaxseed Oil
- Hemp Oil
- Coconut Oil
- Coconut Butter
- Coconut Cream; concentrated, natural

Proteins

- Beef
- Lamb
- Veal
- Goat
- Wild recreation
- Pork
- Hen
- Turkey
- Duck
- Goose
- Sport birds
- Anchovies
- Crab
- Cod
- Catfish
- Calamari
- Flounder
- Halibut
- Mackerel
- Herring
- Mahi-mahi
- Salmon; canned
- Scallops
- Scrod
- Snapper
- Sole
- Tuna - canned is allowed
- Trout

- Lobster
- Squid
- Shrimp
- Mussels

- Oysters
- Complete eggs
- Peanut Butter
- Tempeh

- Tofu
- Edamame
- Whey protein powders

Greens

- Alfalfa sprouts
- Avocado
- Asparagus
- Bamboo shoots
- Beet greens
- Bean sprouts
- Bok choy
- Brussels sprouts
- Bell peppers *
- Broccoli
- Cabbage
- Cauliflower
- Carrots *
- Celery
- Chard

- Celery root
- Chives
- Collard greens
- Cucumbers
- Dandelion greens
- Pickles; dill
- Garlic
- Kale
- Leeks
- Arugula
- Boston butter lettuce
- Endive
- Chicory
- Fennel
- Escarole

- Radicchio
- Romaine
- Mushrooms
- Olives
- Onions *
- Radishes
- Sauerkraut
- Scallions
- Shallots
- Snow peas
- Spinach
- Summer time squash *
- Tomatoes *
- Turnips
- Zucchini

- Water   chestnuts

* These greens are larger in carbohydrates so consumption ought to be restricted.

Dairy Products

- Heavy whipping cream
- Bitter cream; full fats, learn labels for Ingredients and fillers
- Cottage cheese; full fat
- Swiss Cheddar
- Colby
- Monterey Jack
- Provolone
- Munster
- Gouda
- Farmer cheese
- Blue cheese
- Cream cheese
- Mascarpone
- Yogurt; unsweetened, full fats
- Greek yogurt, restrict how a lot you eat as a result of larger carb content material

Nuts & Seeds

- Macadamias
- Pecans
- Almonds
- Walnuts
- Cashews
- Pistachios
- Chestnuts
- Almond flour
- Peanuts
- Pumpkin seeds
- Sunflower seeds
- Sesame seeds
- Hemp seeds
- Chia seeds

Remove any anti-vitamins by soaking or roasting the nuts and seeds. Keep in mind that they are very high in carbs. Eating too many can cause irritation and trigger a disruption in your mood.

Drinks

- Water
- Flavored seltzer water
- Bone broth
- Decaffeinated espresso
- Decaffeinated tea
- Natural tea
- Lemon juice
- Lime juice
- Almond milk
- Hazelnut milk
- Cashew milk
- Coconut milk
- Soy milk
- Hemp milk

*All drinks must be unsweetened

Fruits, Spices & Others

- Blueberries
- Strawberries
- Raspberries
- Cranberries
- Blackberries

- Basil
- Bay leaves
- Black pepper
- Cayenne pepper
- Cardamom
- Cilantro
- Cinnamon
- Chili powder
- Cumin
- Ginger
- Oregano
- Parsley
- Sage
- Thyme
- Rosemary
- Turmeric

*Most fruits contain excessive carbohydrates while some berries may be consumed in small quantities.

Any spice that you don't grind your self will include carbohydrates. Commercially made spice mixes normally include added sugar.

For salting dishes, use sea_salt moderately.

There are web sites that can help you put in your full recipe, together with spices, and the location will calculate your whole macros in addition to energy which can show you how to embody these 'negligible' carbs.

Different gadgets you possibly can get pleasure from in restricted quantities are Japanese Shirataki noodles, pork rinds and eighty five-ninety% chocolate. Pork rinds are a great substitute for bread crumbs however they're excessive in protein so it is best to restrict your use of them.

Some ketogenic recipes, especially desserts, require some sweetening and you actually ought to be cautious about how a lot synthetic sweetener you utilize since you are attempting to get an extra pure eating regimen going. That being mentioned, one of the best sweeteners to make use of is pure like honey or agave. You simply have to be very cautious about how a lot you utilize and comply with the recipe precisely so that you're not including too many carbohydrates to your each day allotment.

Foods You Should Avoid

Sugars & Sweeteners

- Maple syrup
- Malt syrup
- Treacle
- Carob syrup
- Brown sugar
- Turbinado sugar
- White sugar
- Confectioner's or powdered sugar
- Beet sugar
- Cane juice
- Cane syrup
- Caramel
- Panela
- Panocha
- Coconut sugar
- Date sugar
- Corn syrup
- Sorghum
- Molasses
- Rice syrup
- Maltose
- Barley malt
- Maltodextrin
- Fruit syrups
- Fruit juice concentrate
- Tapioca syrup
- Any food that ends in -ose.

Grains & Grain Products

- Wheat
- Barley
- Oats
- Rye
- Sorghum
- Tricale
- Spelt
- Rice
- Bread
- Muffins
- Rolls
- Bread crumbs
- Waffles
- Pancakes
- Pasta
- Any commercial cereals; hot and cold
- Tortillas
- Crackers
- Cookies
- Tarts
- Cakes
- Pies
- Pretzels

- Oatmeal
- Cous Cous
- Cream of wheat
- Quinoa
- Kashi

- Cornbread
- Tamale wrappers
- Corn chips
- Grits

- Polenta
- Popcorn
- Cornmeal

Fruits, Vegetables & Legumes

- Apples
- Bananas
- Plantains
- Pears
- Oranges
- Grapefruits
- Peaches
- Apricots
- Currents
- Cantaloupe
- Honeydew
- Melon
- Watermelon
- Cherries
- Dates
- Figs
- Gooseberries

- Grapes
- Raisins
- Guava
- Mango
- Nectarines
- Kiwi
- Papaya
- Plums
- Pineapple
- Pumpkin
- Pomegranates
- Potatoes
- Sweet potatoes
- Hash browns
- Potato chips
- Tater tots
- French fries

- Mashed potatoes
- Corn
- Lima beans
- Peas
- Okra
- Artichokes
- Kidney beans
- Black beans
- Black-eyed peas
- Chickpeas
- Great northern beans
- Vegetable juice concentrate
- Lentil

Other Foods You Should Avoid:

- Canned soups

- Canned stews

- Processed, boxed 'convenience' foods

- Foods listed as 'low-fat', 'low-carb', 'sugar-free', etc.

- Beer

- Hard liquor

- Sweet or dessert wines; dry wines are allowed in limited amounts

- Carbonated drinks, diet and non-diet

- Milk; any liquid milk that contains lactose.

Finding Meal Plans That Will Fit Your Life

Finding a meal plan that will fit your lifestyle is quite easy to do. With an abundance of websites offering ready-made meal plans and thousands of recipes, you will never have a hard time figuring out what to eat with the ketogenic diet.

Now that you have your daily percentages and the recommended grams, here are a few other things that you should consider for a successful ketogenic lifestyle.

Here is a 7 Step Guide on how to create a Keto Meal Plan:

1. Draft – Consider the foods you like to eat on the approved list and draft your own ketogenic diet plan. Remember, the ketogenic diet included high-fat, moderate protein and low-carbs.

2. Check – Check the recipes in your meal plan and see if the fats, proteins, and carbs match up to your body weight. If not, readjust your mean plan.

3. Research – Before you start your meal plan, research other methods of the keto diet plan and see how they compare. Be sure to complete this guide as you don't want to jump into this head first.

4. Revise – Revise any changes that should be made and improve recipes that could be better.

5. Converse – Talk with a ketogenic expert! If you are still unsure, follow our sample meal plan and ask around.

6. Repair – Check for any needed improvement and make the final changes to your diet plan. Make sure it matches your needs of the 75:20:5%

7. Follow Through – Go ahead and get started!

Sample Ketogenic Meal Plan

If you like to keep your meal plan and recipes simple and easy, feel free to use this guide to help get you started. Once you've become more comfortable in the steps of following the ketogenic, use this 7-day Ketogenic mean plan as a reference for your ketogenic meal plan.

	Breakfast	**Lunch**	**Dinner**
Day 1	Keto poppy Seed Lemon Muffins	Coconut Prawns	Avocado and Salmon Stacks
Day 2	2 fried Eggs with 2 strips of Bacon	Tuna and Cucumber Wraps	Maki
Day 3	Keto Breakfast Burger	Paprika Tacos with Guacamole	Roasted Turkey
Day 4	Bacon cheddar Chive omelet	Zucchini Patties with Cauli-bread	Rib eye and Wild mushroom soup
Day 5	Jalapeno Cheddar Waffles	Two hamburger patties with bacon and cheese	Lamb with Okra
Day 6	Keto Cinnamon "Oatmeal"	Two hot dog sausages with simple salad	Mediterranean Meatballs
Day 7	Poached eggs with melted cheese and spinach	Green salad with grated cheese and cubed ham	French Mussels

CHAPTER 5: HOW TO MAKE THE KETOGENIC DIET WORK FOR YOU

Tips for successful transitioning

1. **Cook for yourself** – freeze the remaining servings or save half of the recipes, if needed.

2. **Swap Your Meals** – you can swap your meals anytime of the day. Eat breakfast for lunch or lunch for dinner. Your mean plan depends on you!

3. **Make Keto Buns in advance** – bake the Keto buns in batches and place them in a freezer to keep them fresh. Defrost overnight at room temperature or place in the oven before serving.

4. **Try to Skip the Snacks** – While you should feel satisfied from the 3 main meals, keep Keto-friendly snacks close by.

5. **Understand that diet plans are not suitable for everyone** – Make sure that your daily requirements match your recipes and diet plan. Make small adjustments and reduce the portions if needed. Don't worry if you go over your protein intake a bit, as it will not kick you out of ketosis and will actually keep hunger at bay. If you find yourself lacking enough fat in your diet, add more fat by adding oils and fatty foods according to your adjustments.

6. **Only eat when hungry** – if you don't feel hunger, don't eat.

7. **It's OKAY to Substitute** – fish, pork, and lamb can be substituted with one another in recipes due to their similar nutritional value.

Dining out and Enjoying Snacks!

Having a Snack

While most people following the ketogenic diet do perfectly well with 2-3 meals a day, others may need snacks in order to maintain feeling satisfied and staying in ketosis. Be sure to include snacks into your meal plan if you must. Have a snack every two hours to keep your system running at tip-top shape. Here is a list of healthy snacks to give you a boost:

- Boiled eggs
- Cheeses
- Sliced ham
- Cream cheese roll-ups
- Olives
- Nuts
- Canned sardines
- Leftover meat
- Shrimp; boiled or steams
- Avocado
- Sugarless beef jerky
- Tuna salad with cucumber

If you find yourself feeling hungry between meals, this may be due to the lack of fat and protein in your diet.

In the Restaurant

Yes, you CAN still eat out while following the ketogenic lifestyle. While this doesn't mean you should eat less, you must eat intelligently and know the approved food list to keep in mind as you order. In the beginning, you may feel that the ketogenic diet isn't that easy when you are invited to eat out.

To save you from stressing over what to order, simply choose fish or meat for the main dish and opt for vegetables and salad instead of rice or bread. Ask for extra butter to spread onto your vegetables or steak to add more flavor and moisture. Request for olive or coconut oil as well.

If you're going to a fast food place or a sports bar, chicken wings and hamburgers are the least bad option even with the extra sauces on the wings. Obviously, be sure to avoid fries and soft drinks. But add lemon to your water, even when friends are indulging in beer.

With that being said, the more you follow the ketogenic diet every day, the less eating out will become an issue. If the events that you are unsure of the menu or visiting a friend's home for a meal, eat something at home before you leave. This will allow you to limit portions and refrain from foods you shouldn't eat.

CHAPTER 6: KETOGENIC RECIPES

BREAKFAST RECIPES

KETO POPPY SEED LEMON MUFFINS

Ingredients

- 2 large Eggs
- 3/4 cup Almond Flour
- 1/3 cup Erythritol Powder
- 1/4 cup Flaxseed Meal
- 1/4 cup Heavy Cream
- 1/4 cup Salted Butter -melted
- 3 tbsp. Lemon Juice
- 2 tbsp. Poppy Seeds
- 1 tsp. Baking Powder
- 1 tsp. Vanilla Extract
- Zest of 2 Lemons

Directions

1. Pre-heat oven to 350 F.

2. In a mixing bowl, combine erythritol, flaxseed meal, almond flour, and poppy seeds together.

3. Add in the eggs, melted butter, and heavy cream and stir until smooth. Then add the baking powder, vanilla, lemon juice, and lemon zest. Mix until well combined.

4. Pour the batter equally into 12 cupcake molds and bake for 18-20 minutes or until golden brown. Remove from heat and let cool for about 10 minutes.

5. Slice and serve immediately!

Each serving contains:

129 Calories, 11.3g Fats, 1.5g Net Carbs, and 3.7g Protein.

KETO CON HUEVOS

Ingredients

- 3 Eggs

- 2 slices Bacon

- 1 Jalapeno Pepper - de-seeded

- 1 Avocado

- 1 Tomato

- 1/4 medium Onion

- 1 oz. Pork Rinds

- 1/4 cup Cilantro, chopped

- Salt and Pepper, to Taste

Directions

1. Pour cold water over bacon then fry until cooked. Remove from heat and place on paper towels. Keep the fat in the pan.

2. Cook the pork rinds in bacon fat then add the vegetables. When the onions are translucent, begin to stir in the cilantro. Add the scrambled eggs and cook, stirring once.

3. Cube the avocado and combine with the dish.

4. Serve immediately and enjoy!

Each serving contains :
254 Calories, 21.5g Fats, 2.5g Net Carbs, and 12.4g Protein.

KETO BREAKFAST BURGER

Ingredients

- 4 slices Bacon
- 2 large Eggs
- 4 oz. Sausage
- 2 oz. Pepper jack Cheese
- 1 tbsp. Butter
- Salt and Pepper, to Taste

Directions

1. Preheat oven at 400 F.

2. Cook bacon in the oven for 20-25 minutes. Add the butter and set aside.

3. Cook the sausage patties on both sides. Add cheese, and cover with a lid. Remove from pan. Cook egg over easy and place on top.

4. Serve immediately and enjoy!

Each serving contains

654.5 Calories, 55.9g Fats, 3g Net Carbs, and 30.4g Protein

JALAPENO CHEDDAR WAFFLES

Ingredients

- 3 large Eggs
- 1 small Jalapeno
- 3 oz. Cream Cheese
- 1 oz. Cheddar Cheese
- 1 tbsp. Coconut Flour
- 1 tsp. Psyllium Husk Powder
- 1 tsp. Baking Powder
- Salt and Pepper, to taste

Directions

1. Mix all the ingredients together using a blender, until everything is smooth.

2. Prepare your waffle iron, and then pour the waffle mix. Top with your favorite toppings.

3. Serve immediately and enjoy!

Each serving contains 337 Calories, 27g Fats, 3g Net Carbs, and 15.9g Protein.

BACON CHEDDAR CHIVE OMELET

Ingredients

- 2 slices Bacon, already cooked
- 2 large Eggs
- 2 stalks Chives
- 1 oz. Cheddar Cheese
- 1 tsp. Bacon Fat
- Salt and Pepper, to taste

Directions

1. Prepare all ingredients and heat pan to a medium-low with bacon fat. Add the eggs, and season with chives, salt, and pepper.

2. As soon as the edges begin to set, add bacon to the middle and cook for 20-30 seconds and remove from heat.

3. Top with cheese and fold the edges on top like a burrito. Flip over and warm through on the other side.

4. Serve immediately and enjoy!

Each serving contains 462 Calories, 40g Fats, 1g Net Carbs, and 23g Protein.

KETO PEANUT PANCAKES

Ingredients

- Peanut Filling
- 2 oz. Fresh Peanuts
- 1/2 tsp. Stevia
- Salt, to taste

Condensed Milk

- 1/4 cup Heavy Cream
- 2 drops Liquid Sucralose

Apam Balik

- 1 large Egg
- 1/2 cup Almond Flour
- 1/4 cup Almond Milk
- 1 tbsp. Unsalted Butter
- 1/2 tsp. Bicarbonate Soda
- 1/2 tsp. Baking Powder
- 1/2 tsp. Vanilla Extract
- 1/4 tsp. Coconut Oil
- 1/8 tsp. Salt
- 4-5 drops Liquid Sucralose

Directions

1. Roast peanuts until browned. Grind the peanuts with salt and stevia, to taste.

2. Heat the liquid sucralose and heavy cream until thickened. Mix the almond flour, baking powder, baking soda and salt. Add the egg, almond milk, liquid sucralose and vanilla extract and mix until well-combined.

3. In a heated pan, melt half of the coconut oil and pour in the mixture. Cover for 1 minute. Sprinkle half of the ground peanuts and spread half of the Keto condensed milk and butter.

4. Cover the pan until cooked and remove the pancake to let it cool.

5. Repeat until mixture is cooked. Serve immediately and enjoy!

Each serving contains 389 Calories, 38.9g Fats, 3.8g Net Carbs, and 13.5g Protein.

LOW-CARB KETO PAN SANDWICH

Ingredients

Pancake Buns

- 1/3 oz. Pork rings
- 1 egg – beaten
- 2 tbsp. Keto maple syrup
- 1 tbsp. Almond flour
- 1 tbsp. heavy cream

Filling

- 2 oz. Sausage
- 1 Egg
- 1 slice Cheddar Cheese

Directions

1. In heated pan, place the sausage in a ring bold and cook the sausage until medium-well. Set aside in foil once cooked.

2. Place the pork rinds in a food processor and grind until powder is formed, then mix altogether with the bun ingredients.

3. Add 1/2 batter onto the ring mold and cook on each side until browned. Remove the mold and flip over. Repeat until mixture is cooked.

4. Add the egg to the mold. Allow to cook until solidified. Assemble the sandwich with cheese, egg, and sausage.

5. Serve immediately and enjoy!

Each serving contains 657 Calories, 55.7g Fats, 2.7g Net Carbs, and 40g Protein.

PUMPKIN BREAD

Ingredients

- 3 large Egg Whites
- 1 1/2 cup Almond Flour
- 1 1/2 tsp. Pumpkin Pie Spice
- 1/2 cup Pumpkin Puree
- 1/2 cup Coconut Milk
- 1/4 cup Psyllium Husk Powder
- 1/4 cup Stevia
- 2 tsp Baking Powder
- 1/2 tsp. Salt

Directions

1. Preheat oven to 350 F. Place a container with 1 cup of water on the bottom rack.

2. Mix all the dry ingredients into a mixing bowl and add the pumpkin ingredients and coconut milk into dry ingredients. Mix well until combined. Whip the egg whites until stiff and slowly fold the egg whites into dough.

3. Spread the dough onto a greased loaf pan, and then place the mixture into the oven. Bake for 75 minutes. Let the bread load cool then slice into serving pieces.

3. Serve immediately and enjoy!

Each serving contains 120 Calories, 8.7g Fats, 3.1g Net Carbs, and 4.5g Protein.

SPICED PUMPKIN FRENCH TOAST

Ingredients

- 4 slices Pumpkin Bread (refer to recipe above)
- 1 large Egg
- 2 tbsp. Butter
- 2 tbsp. Cream
- 1/2 tsp. Vanilla Extract
- 1/4 tsp. Pumpkin Pie Spice
- 1/8 tsp. Orange Extract

Directions

1. Allow the bread to dry out overnight in open air. Mix the pumpkin pie spice, egg, and extracts together. Place the bread into the mixture and let the pumpkin mixture each loaf soak on both sides.

2. Heat the butter in a pan, and then add the marinated slices. Flip over and cook until browned on each side.

3. Top with Keto maple syrup and Enjoy!

Each serving contains 428 Calories, 37.4g Fats, 6.8g Net Carbs, and 12g Protein.

KETO CINNAMON OATMEAL

Ingredients

- 3 1/2 cups Coconut Milk
- 1 cup Crushed Pecans
- 3 oz. Cream Cheese
- 1/2 cup Cauliflower, riced
- 1/3 cup Flax Seed
- 1/3 cup Chia Seed
- 1/4 cup Heavy Cream
- 3 tbsp. Butter
- 3 tbsp. Erythritol powder
- 1/2 tbsp. Cinnamon
- 1/2 tbsp. Maple Flavor
- 1/2 tsp. Vanilla
- 1/4 tsp. All spice
- 1/4 tsp. Nutmeg
- 10-15 drops Liquid Stevia

Directions

1. Prepare the rice cauliflower in a food processor and set aside. Heat the coconut milk in a pan over medium heat. Crush the pecans and add to the pan over low-heat until toasted.

2. Add the cauliflower to coconut milk and bring to a boil. Reduce to a simmer and stir in the spices and mix until well-combined. Add the Erythritol powder to the pan. Add the stevia, flax, and chia seeds.

3. Lastly, add the butter, cream and cream cheese to the pan and mix again.

4. Serve immediately and enjoy!

Each serving contains 359 Calories, 30.4g Fats, 5g Net Carbs, and 9.4g Protein.

MAIN RECIPES

AVOCADO, CHICKEN AND BACON SANDWICH

Ingredients

Keto Cloud Bread

- 3 large Eggs
- 3 oz. Cream Cheese
- 1/2 tsp. Garlic Powder
- 1/4 tsp. Salt
- 1/8 tsp. Cream of Tartar

Filling

- 1/4 medium Avocado - mashed
- 3 oz. Chicken
- 2 Grape Tomatoes
- 2 slices Bacon
- 2 slices Pepper Jack Cheese
- 1 tbsp. Mayonnaise
- 1 tsp. Sriracha

Directions

1. Preheat the oven to 300F.

2. Place 3 eggs into separate bowls. Add salt and cream of tartar to the egg whites, then whip until soft and foamy results.

3. In the other bowl, beat yolks and cream cheese. Gently fold the egg whites into the yolk mixture. On a parchment paper lined baking sheet, spoon 1/4 cup of the batter, then form into squares. Sprinkle the garlic over the top and bake for 25 minutes.

4. Cook the chicken and bacon with salt and pepper to taste. Assemble the sandwich with mayo, sriracha, tomatoes, cheese, and mashed avocado.

Each serving contains 361 Calories, 28.3g Fats, 2g Net Carbs, and 22g Protein.

AVOCADO TUNA MELT BITES

Ingredients

- 1 (10 oz.) Can Tuna, drained
- 1 medium Avocado, cubed
- 1/2 cup Coconut Oil, for frying
- 1/3 cup Almond Flour
- 1/4 cup Parmesan Cheese
- 1/4 cup Mayonnaise
- 1/2 tsp. Garlic Powder
- 1/2 tsp. Onion Powder
- Salt and Pepper, to Taste

Directions

1. Add all ingredients, except the avocado and coconut oil into a bowl and mix.

2. Cut the avocado into cubes and fold into the tuna. Form the tuna into balls and cover with almond flour.

3. Heat the coconut oil in a pan over medium heat. Once hot, add the tuna balls and fry until browned.

4. Serve immediately and enjoy!

Each bite contains 135 Calories, 11.8g Fats, 0.8g Net Carbs, and 6.2g Protein.

CHEESE STUFFED BACON HOT DOGS

Ingredients

- 12 slices of Bacon
- 6 Hot Dogs
- 2 oz. Cheddar Cheese
- 1/2 tsp. Onion Powder
- 1/2 tsp. Garlic Powder
- Salt and Pepper, to Taste

Directions

1. Pre-heat oven to 400 F.

2. Make a slit in each hot dog and insert sliced cheese into the slits. Wrap each hot dog in 2 slices of bacon each, then secure bacon with toothpicks.

3. Place hot dogs on of a cookie sheet, then season the hot dogs. Bake for 35-40 minutes until golden. Serve immediately and enjoy!

Each hot dog contains 380 Calories, 34.5g Fats, 0.3g Net Carbs, and 16.8g Protein.

ZUCCHINI BROCCOLI CHICKEN SLIDERS

Ingredients

- 2 large zucchinis - hallowed out
- 6 oz. Rotisserie Chicken, shredded
- 3 oz. Cheddar Cheese, shredded
- 1 stalk Green Onion
- 1 cup Broccoli
- 2 tbsp. Sour Cream
- 2 tbsp. Butter – melted
- Salt and Pepper, to taste

Directions

1. Preheat the oven to 400 F.

2. Cut the zucchini in half lengthwise and scoop out most of the zucchini until you're left with a shell about 1cm thick. Pour the butter into each zucchini. Season with salt and pepper. Place the zucchini in the oven and bake for about 20 minutes.

3. While the zucchini is cooking, shred the chicken. Cut the broccoli florets into small pieces and combine with sour cream. Season with salt and pepper.

4. Once the zucchini is done, add the chicken and broccoli filling. Sprinkle cheddar cheese on each zucchini boat and bake for another 10-15 minutes or until the cheese is melted.

5. Garnish with chopped green onion and enjoy with Keto mayo. Serve immediately and enjoy!

Each serving contains 33.9g Fats, 5g Net Carbs, and 29.9g Protein.

KETO HAM AND CHEESE STROMBOLI

Ingredients

- 4 oz. Ham
- 3.5 oz. Cheddar Cheese
- 1 large Egg
- 1 1/4 cups Mozzarella Cheese, shredded
- 4 tbsp. Almond Flour
- 3 tbsp. Coconut Flour
- 1 tsp. Italian Seasoning
- Salt and Pepper, to taste

Directions

1. Preheat oven to 400 F.

2. In a microwave, melt the mozzarella cheese on low heat for about 1 minute, then 10 second intervals, stirring occasionally until melted.

3. Combine the coconut flour, almond flour and seasonings in a mixing bowl, then place the melted mozzarella on top and begin working it in. After a minute, add the egg and combine everything together. Once everything is combined, transfer it to a flat surface and lay a sheet of parchment paper on top.

4. Use a rolling pin or your hand to flatten it out. Cut in diagonal lines leaving a row of dough untouched about 4 inches wide. Alternate laying the ham and cheddar on that uncut dough. Then lift one section of the cut dough and lay it over the top, covering your filling.

5. Bake for 15-20 minutes, until golden. Serve immediately and enjoy!

Each serving contains 306 Calories, 21.8g Fats, 4.7g Net Carbs, and 25.6g Protein.

LOW-CARB PEPPER AND SAUSAGE SOUP

Ingredients

- 32 oz. Pork Sausage
- 10 oz. Raw Spinach
- 1 can Tomatoes w/ Jalapenos
- 1 medium Green Bell Pepper
- 4 cups Beef Stock
- 1 tbsp. Olive Oil
- 1 tbsp. Chili powder
- 1 tbsp. Cumin
- 1 tsp. Italian Seasoning
- 1 tsp. Onion Powder
- 1 tsp. Garlic Powder
- Salt and pepper, to taste

Directions

1. Heat olive oil in a large pot over medium heat. Add the sausage.

2. Slice the green peppers, then add to the pot. Stir until well-combined and season with salt and pepper. Add the jalapenos and tomatoes and continue to stir. Then add the spinach and place the lid on the pot.

3. Add the broth and spices and mix together. Cook for 30 minutes covered, reducing heat to medium-low. Remove the lid from the pan and let simmer for 15 minutes.

4. Serve immediately and enjoy!

Each serving contains 526 Calories, 43g Fats, 3.8g Net Carbs, and 27.8g Protein

KETO EGG DROP SOUP

Ingredients

- 2 large Eggs
- 1 1/2 cups Chicken Broth
- ½ Chicken Bouillon cube
- 1 tbsp. Butter
- 1 tsp. Chili Garlic Paste

Directions

1. Heat pan over medium-high heat. Add the chicken broth, bouillon cube, and or butter to the pan.

2. Bring the broth to a boil, add the chili garlic paste and continue to stir. Remove from heat. Mix the eggs and gently pour into the simmering broth, stirring occasionally.

3. Serve immediately and enjoy!

Each serving contains 279 Calories, 23g Fats, 2.5g Net Carbs, and 12g Protein.

LOW-CARB LIME CHILI MEATBALLS

Ingredients

For the Meatballs

- 1 lb. Ground Chicken
- 2 medium Spring Onions, chopped
- 1/2 medium Red Bell Pepper
- 1/2 Lime, juiced and zest
- 2 oz. Cheddar Cheese
- 2 tbsps. Flaxseed Meal
- 2 tbsps. Almond Flour
- 2 tbsp. Cilantro, chopped
- 1 tsp. Garlic Powder
- 1 tsp. Red Pepper Flakes
- Salt

Guacamole

- 1 medium Avocado – mashed
- 1/2 medium Lime juice
- 1/4 tsp. Garlic Powder
- Salt & Pepper, to Taste

Directions

1. Preheat oven to 350 F.

2. Shred the Cheddar Cheese and set aside in a bowl. Prepare all the vegetables and add to the ground chicken. Chop 2 tbsp. cilantro and add to the bowl.

3. Season with spices and lime juice into the chicken meatball mixture and add the lime zest. Add the flaxseed meal and almond flour. Mix until well-combined.

4. Roll meatballs and bake for 15-18 minute, until cooked.

5. Prepare the guacamole: Mash the avocado, lime juice, garlic powder together. Add salt and pepper to taste.

6. Serve immediately and enjoy!

Each serving contains 428 Calories, 31.3g Fats, 4.7g Net Carbs, and 33.7g Protein.

BBQ-STYLE CHICKEN SOUP

Ingredients

Soup Base

- 3 medium Chicken Thighs
- 1 1/2 cup Beef Broth
- 1 1/2 cup Chicken Broth
- 2 tbsp. Olive Oil
- 2 tsp. Chili Seasoning
- Salt and Pepper, to Taste

BBQ Sauce

- 1/4 Cup Keto Ketchup
- 1/4 cup Tomato Paste
- 1/4 cup Butter
- 2 tbsp. Dijon Mustard
- 1 tbsp. Soy Sauce
- 1 tbsp. hot sauce
- 2 1/2 tsp. Liquid Smoke
- 1 1/2 tsp. Garlic Powder
- 1 tsp. Worcestershire Sauce
- 1 tsp. Red Chili Flakes
- 1 tsp. Onion Powder
- 1 tsp. Cumin
- 1 tsp. Chili Powder

Directions

1. Preheat oven to 400 F.

2. Remove the bone from the chicken thighs, and set aside. Season with your favorite chili seasoning. Place on a baking tray with foil and bake for 50 minutes.

3. Meanwhile, add the Olive Oil in a pot over medium-high heat. Once hot, add the chicken bones. Allow to cook for 5 minutes and the add broths. Season with salt and pepper to taste.

4. Once the chicken is done, remove the skins and set aside. Add all of the fat from the chicken thighs into the broth and stir.

5. To make the BBQ sauce: Combine the ingredients above and mix well. Add the bbq sauce to the pot and stir together. Allow to simmer for 20-30 minutes. Shred the chicken thighs and add to the soup. Simmer for another 10-20 minutes. Serve with cheddar cheese, yellow bell pepper, spring onion and crispy chicken skins.

6. Serve immediately and enjoy!

Each serving contains 486 Calories, 38g Fats, 4.2g Net Carbs, and 24.6g Protein.

SOUTHWESTERN PORK STEW

Ingredients

- 1 lb. Cooked Pork Shoulder, sliced
- 6 oz. Button Mushrooms
- 1/2 Jalapeno – sliced
- 1/2 Onion
- 1/2 Green Bell Pepper - sliced
- 1/2 Red Bell Pepper - sliced
- 2 cups Gelatinous Bone Broth
- 2 cup Chicken Broth
- 1/2 cup Strong Coffee
- 1/4 cup Tomato Paste
- 2 Bay Leaves
- 2 tsp. Chili Powder
- 2 tsp. Cumin
- 1 tsp. Paprika
- 1 tsp. Oregano
- 1 tsp. Minced Garlic
- 1/2 tsp. Salt
- 1/2 tsp. Pepper
- 1/4 tsp. Cinnamon
- 1/2 Lime - juice

Directions

1. Prepare vegetables. Sauté vegetables in a pan over high-heat in olive oil. Once aromatic, remove from heat.

2. Chop pork and add to slow cooker. Add the bone broth, mushrooms, chicken broth, and coffee. Add the spices and vegetables to the slow cooker. Mix until well-combined. Replace lid and cook on low for 4-10 hours.

3. Serve and enjoy!

Each serving contains 386 Calories, 28.9g Fats, 6.4g Net Carbs, and 19.9g Protein.

SPICED PUMPKIN SOUP

Ingredients

- 4 slices Bacon
- 1 cup Pumpkin Puree
- 1.5 cups Chicken Broth
- 1/2 cup Heavy Cream
- 1/4 Onion - chopped
- 4 tbsp. Butter
- 2 cloves Garlic - minced
- 1 Bay Leaf
- 1/2 tsp. Freshly Minced Ginger
- 1/2 tsp. Pepper
- 1/4 tsp. Cinnamon
- 1/4 tsp. Coriander
- 1/8 tsp. Nutmeg
- Salt
- 3 tbsp. Bacon Grease – for frying

Directions

1. Brown butter in a saucepan over low heat. Add the onions, garlic, and ginger to the pan and cook for 2-3 minutes.

2. Once onions are translucent, add the spices and stir well. Allow to cook for 1-2 minutes, then add pumpkin and chicken broth into the pan.

3. Bring the mixture to boil, then reduce to low heat. Allow to simmer for 20 minutes. Place the mixture in a blender to puree until smooth. Return the mixture to the pan and allow to simmer for another 20 minutes.

4. Meanwhile, cook 4 slices of bacon.

5. Once the soup is done, add the heavy cream and bacon grease and mix. Crumble bacon over the top and add chopped parsley and 2 tbsp. sour cream.

6. Serve immediately and enjoy!

THAI SHRIMP CURRY

Ingredients

- 6 oz. Pre-cooked Shrimp
- 5 oz. Broccoli Florets
- 1 medium Spring Onion, chopped
- 1 cup Vegetable Stock
- 1 cup Coconut Milk
- 1/2 cup Sour Cream - for topping
- 3 tbsp. Cilantro, chopped
- 2 tbsp. Green Curry Paste
- 2 tbsp. Coconut Oil
- 1 tbsp. Peanut Butter
- 1 tbsp. Soy Sauce
- 1/2 Lime Juice
- 1 tsp. Crushed Roasted Garlic
- 1 tsp. Fish Sauce
- 1 tsp. Minced Ginger
- 1/2 tsp. Turmeric
- 1/4 tsp. Xanthan Gum

Directions

1. Add coconut oil to a pan over medium heat. Add the ginger, garlic, and chopped spring onion.

2. Allow the ingredients to cook, then add green curry paste, fish sauce, turmeric, soy sauce and peanut butter. Stir well, then add vegetable broth and coconut milk. Add 1/4 tsp. xanthan gum and mix.

3. Allow the curry to thicken. Add the broccoli and stir in well. Chop the cilantro and add to the pan.

4. Lastly, add the shrimp and mix everything together. Allow to cook for a few minutes, then serve with sour cream. Enjoy!

Each serving contains 455 Calories, 31.5g Fats, 8.9g Net Carbs, and 27g Protein.

KETO GRILLED CHEESE

Ingredients

Bun Ingredients

- 2 whole Eggs
- 2 tbsp. Butter
- 2 tbsps. Almond Flour
- 1 tbsp. Psyllium Husk Powder
- 1/2 tsp. Baking Powder

Fillings

- 2 Oz. Cheddar Cheese
- 1 tbsp. Butter - for frying

Directions

1. Combine the bun ingredients together in a container. Pour the mixture into a square bowl or container. Place the bowl in the microwave and cook for 90 seconds. Continue to check if it's done. If not, continue every 15 seconds until cooked.

2. Remove bread from the container and slice in half. Place the cheese between the buns. Heat the butter in a pan over medium heat, then fry the grilled cheese.

3. Serve immediately and enjoy!

1 serving contains 793 Calories, 70g Fats, 4.7g Net Carbs, and 29g Protein.

FRESH BASIL BELL PEPPER PIZZA

Ingredients

Pizza Base

- 6 oz. Mozzarella Cheese
- 1 large Egg
- ½ cup Almond Flour
- 2 tbsps. Parmesan Cheese
- 2 tbsps. Psyllium Husk
- 2 tbsps. Cream Cheese
- 1 tsp. Italian Seasoning
- Salt and Pepper, to taste

Toppings

- 1 medium Vine Tomato
- 4 oz. Shredded Cheddar Cheese
- 1/4 cup Rao's Tomato Sauce
- 2/3 medium Bell Pepper
- 2-3 tbsp. Fresh Chopped Basil

Directions

1. Preheat oven to 400 F.

2. Microwave the mozzarella cheese for 40 seconds or until completely melted. Add the rest of the pizza ingredients to the cheese and mix together well with your hands. (Except the toppings)

3. Using your hands or a rolling pin, flatten the dough and form a circle. Allow to bake for 10 minutes, and remove pizza from the oven. Top the pizza with the toppings and bake for another 10 minutes. Remove pizza from the oven and let cool.

4. Serve immediately and enjoy!

KETO STEAK FAJITAS

Ingredients

Filling

- 3 medium Jalapenos
- 2 lbs. Skirt Steak
- 1 medium Bell Pepper
- 1 small Red Chili Pepper
- 1 small Onion
- 1/2 can Whole Tomatoes
- 3 tbsp. Ketchup
- 1 tbsp. Apple Cider Vinegar
- 2 tsp. Cumin
- 1 tsp. Liquid Smoke
- 1 tsp. Minced Garlic
- Salt & Pepper, to taste

Tortillas

- 1/2 cup Chicken or Beef Broth
- 1/4 cup Coconut Flour
- 2 tbsp. Butter
- 1 tbsp. Ground Psyllium Husk
- 1 pinch Garlic Powder
- 1 pinch Seasoning Salt

Directions

1. Remove skin from skirt steak. Prepare and cut all vegetables into bite-size pieces. Remove seeds from the jalapenos and red chili.

2. Add all ingredients to the crock pot –in layers of vegetables, meat, and another layer of vegetables. Cook on low heat for 6-8 hours.

3. Prepare the tortillas by boiling the broth and mixing it into the other tortilla ingredients. Form the dough and cut small circles.

4. Fry the circles in a pan on the stove over medium-low heat until brown. Add fillings.

5. Serve immediately and enjoy!

Each serving contains 521 Calories, 30.2g Fats, 9.5g Net Carbs, and 36.8g Protein.

SESAME GINGER GLAZED SALMON

Ingredients

- 10 oz. Salmon Filet
- 2 tbsps. White Wine
- 2 Tbsps. Soy Sauce
- 1 tbsp. Red Boat Fish Sauce
- 1 Tbsp. Rice Vinegar
- 1 tbsp. Ketchup
- 1 1/2 tsps. Sesame Oil
- 2 tsps. Minced Garlic
- 1 tsp. Minced Ginger

Directions

1. Add the ingredients except for the sesame oil, ketchup and white wine to a small container. Marinade the ingredients in the liquids for about 10 minutes.

2. Bring a pan to high heat and add the sesame oil. Add the salmon fish skin side down. Allow the fish to cook and skin crisp, then flip and cook on the other side - about 4 minutes per side, depending on thickness. Add the marinate liquids to the pan and let it boil with the fish.

3. Remove fish from pan and set aside. Add the ketchup and white wine to marinate liquids. Let simmer for 5 minutes.

4. Serve immediately and enjoy!

Each serving contains 370 Calories, 23.5g Fats, 2.5g Net Carbs, and 33g Protein.

LOW-CARB MOROCCAN MEATBALLS

Ingredients

Meatballs

- 1 pound ground lamb
- 1 tbsp. Finely Chopped Fresh Cilantro
- 1 tbsp. Finely Chopped Fresh Mint
- 2 tsp. Fresh Thyme
- 1 tsp. Minced Garlic
- 1 tsp. Ground Cumin
- 1 tsp. Ground Coriander
- 1 tsp. Kosher Salt
- 1/2 tsp. Onion Powder
- 1/2 tsp. Allspice
- 1/4 tsp. Oregano
- 1/4 tsp. Curry Powder
- 1/4 tsp. Paprika
- 1/4 tsp. Freshly Ground Black Pepper

Faux Yogurt Sauce

- 1/2 cup Coconut Cream
- 1/2 Lemon zest
- 2 tbsp. Coconut Water
- 1 tbsp. Finely Chopped Fresh Mint
- 1 tbsp. Finely Chopped Fresh Cilantro

- 1 1/4 tsp. Cumin

- 1 tsp. Lemon Juice

- 1/4 tsp. Salt

Directions

1. Preheat oven to 350 F.

2. Combine the ingredients for the meatballs and mix until well-combined. Form 15-18 meatballs and place separately on a foiled baking sheet.

3. Bake for 15-18 minutes or until cooked through. While the meatballs are baking, combine all ingredients for the yogurt sauce and mix thoroughly.

4. Serve immediately and enjoy!

Each serving contains 399 Calories, 32.5g Fats, 3g Net Carbs, and 19.5g Protein.

SEARED STEAL WITH CILANTRO PASTE

Ingredients

Steak Marinade

- 1 lb. Skirt Steak
- 1 medium Lime, juiced
- 1/4 cup Soy Sauce
- 1/4 cup Olive Oil
- 1 small Handful Cilantro
- 1 tsp. Minced Garlic
- 1/4 tsp. Red Pepper Flakes

Cilantro Paste

- 1 medium Jalapeno, seeded
- 1/2 medium Lemon, juiced
- 1 cup Fresh Cilantro, lightly packed
- 1/4 cup Olive Oil
- 1 tsp. Minced Garlic
- ½ tsp. Cumin
- ½ tsp. Coriander
- ½ tsp. Salt

Directions

1. Remove the skin from the skirt steak and add all of the Marinade ingredients to a plastic bag. Marinate the steak for at least 1 hour in the fridge.

2. To make the sauce: Add the Cilantro Paste ingredients to a food processor and pulse until well combined.

3. To cook the steak: Heat a cast iron skillet to medium-high heat. Once hot, add the steak to the pan and cook on each side for about 2-3 minutes per side.

4. Serve immediately and enjoy!

Each serving contains 432 Calories, 32.5g Fats, 1.8g Net Carbs, and 32.3g Protein.

KETO SUSHI

Ingredients

- 16 oz. Cauliflower
- 6 oz. Cream Cheese, softened
- 5 oz. Smoked Salmon, Tuna, Crab or any seafood
- 1/2 medium Avocado
- 1 6 inch Cucumber
- 5 sheets Nori
- 1-2 tbsp. Rice Vinegar
- 1 tbsp. Soy Sauce

Directions

1. Using a food processor, blend cauliflower into riced pieces.

2. Slice the cucumber on each end, then place the cucumber upright and slice off each side. Slice about 2 side pieces into small strips. Set aside.

3. In a heated pan, add cauliflower rice and cook. Season with soy sauce. Once the cauliflower is cooked, add the cauliflower to a bowl with cream cheese and rice vinegar. Mix together well and set in the fridge until cool.

4. Once the rice mixture has cooled down, slice the avocado in half, then into small strips. Place a nori sheet on a bamboo roller covered with saran wrap then spread some the cauliflower rice mixture over the nori sheet, add fillings and roll tightly. Cut into 1 inch slices.

5. Serve immediately and enjoy!

Each serving contains 353 Calories, 25.7g Fats, 5.7g Net Carbs, and 18.3g Protein.

LOW-CARB CHICKEN SATAY

Ingredients

- 1 lb. Ground Chicken
- 2 Spring Onions
- 1/3 Yellow Pepper
- Juice of 1/2 Lime
- 4 Tbsp. Soy Sauce
- 3 Tbsp. Peanut Butter
- 1 Tbsp. Rice Vinegar
- 1 Tbsp. Erythritol
- 2 tsp. Sesame Oil
- 2 tsp. Chili Paste
- 1 tsp. Minced Garlic
- 1/4 tsp. Paprika
- 1/4 tsp. Cayenne

Directions

1. Heat oil in a pan over medium-high heat.

2. Brown the ground chicken, then add all the ingredients. Mix well. Add the chopped spring onions and 1/3 sliced yellow pepper.

3. Serve immediately and enjoy!

Each serving contains 393 Calories, 23g Fats, 3.7g Net Carbs, and 35g Protein.

KETO CHICKEN TIKKA MASALA

Ingredients

- 1 1/2 lbs. Chicken Thighs, with bones and skin
- 1 lb. Chicken Thighs, with bones and skin
- 10 oz. can Diced Tomatoes
- 1 cup Coconut Milk (from the carton)
- 1 cup Heavy Cream
- 1 inch Ginger Root, grated
- 3 cloves Garlic, minced
- 3 tbsp. Tomato Paste
- 2 tbsp. Olive Oil
- 2 tsp. Onion Powder
- 5 tsp. Garam Masala
- 4 tsp. Kosher Salt
- 2 tsp. Smoked Paprika
- 1 tsp. Guar Gum
- Fresh Cilantro

Directions

1. Chop the chicken into bite-sized pieces. Add chicken to the slow cooker and grate 1 inch knob of ginger over the top. Add all dry spices into the slow cooker. Add the tomato paste and diced tomatoes to slow cooker. Mix well.

2. Lastly, add 1/2 cup coconut milk and mix until well-combined. Cook on low for 6 hours or high for 3 hours. Once done, add the heavy cream, coconut milk, and guar gum. Combine well with the chicken.

3. Serve immediately and enjoy!

Each serving contains 492 Calories, 41g Fats, 5.7g Net Carbs, and 25g Protein.

KETO CHILI SOUP

Ingredients

- 16 oz. Chicken Thighs
- 2 oz. Queso Fresco
- 2 Chili Peppers, sliced
- 1 Avocado
- 2 cups Chicken Broth
- 2 cups Water
- 4 tbsp. Tomato Paste
- 2 tbsp. Butter
- 2 tbsp. Olive Oil
- 1 tsp. Turmeric
- 1 tsp. Coriander Seeds
- 1/2 tsp. Ground Cumin
- Juice of half a Lime
- Cilantro
- Salt, Pepper to taste

Directions

1. Prepare the chicken thighs and cook in a heated pan in oil. Set aside.

2. Add olive oil and heat the coriander seeds to release more of their flavor. Add the chili to season the oil. Add the water and broth. Allow to simmer. Season with cumin, turmeric, ground, salt and pepper.

3. Once simmering, add the tomato paste and butter and stir to melt and combine. Let your soup simmer for 5-10 minutes. Add the lime juice.

4. Place the chicken thighs into your bowls and ladle the soup for serving. Garnish with 1/4 of an avocado into each bowl, queso fresco and cilantro.

5. Serve immediately and enjoy!

Each serving comes contains 396 Calories, 27.8g Fats, 5.8g Net Carbs, and 28g Protein.

PUMPKIN CARBONARA

Ingredients

- 1 package Shirataki Noodles
- 5 oz. Pancetta
- 2 large Egg Yolks
- 1/3 cup Parmesan Cheese
- 1/4 cup Heavy Cream
- 3 tbsp. Pumpkin Puree
- 2 tbsp. Butter
- 1/2 tsp. Dried Sage
- Salt and Pepper, to Taste

Directions

1. Rinse off the shirataki noodles under hot water for 2. Dry them off completely and set aside.

2. Chop pancetta and place into a hot pan to sear. Once crisp, remove noodles from the pan and save the fat. Place the butter into a small pot and let brown. Stir in the pumpkin puree and sage. Add pancetta fat and heavy cream to the pumpkin puree sauce and mix until well-combined. Turn the pan to high heat and add the shirataki noodles. Fry them for at least 5 minutes.

3. Add the parmesan cheese to the pumpkin sauce and mix together well. Turn the heat to low and stir until sauce is thickened. Add the noodles and pancetta into the sauce and toss well. Pour the egg yolks and mix into the sauce.

4. Serve immediately and enjoy!

Each serving contains 383 Calories, 34.6g Fats, 2g Net Carbs, and 13g Protein.

KETO KUNG PAO CHICKEN

Ingredients

- 4 red Bird's Eye Chilies, de-seeded
- 2 medium Chicken Thighs, bone in skin on
- 2 large Spring Onions
- 1/2 medium Green Pepper
- 1/4 cup Peanuts
- 1 tsp. Ground Ginger
- Salt and Pepper, to Taste

Sauce

- 2 tbsp. Chili Garlic Paste
- 1 tbsp. Soy Sauce
- 1 tbsp. Ketchup
- 2 tsp. Rice Wine Vinegar
- 2 tsp. Sesame Oil
- 1/2 tsp. Maple Extract
- 10 drops Liquid Stevia

Directions

1. Chop chicken into bite sized pieces and season with salt, pepper, and ginger.

2. Heat the pan over medium-high heat and add the chicken. Cook for 10 minutes. Prepare the vegetables and chili. Set aside.

3. Prepare sauce by combining all ingredients until well combined. Once the chicken is browned, stir everything together and let cook.

4. Add vegetables and peanuts to the pan and cook for 3 minutes. Add the sauce and let it boil to reduce.

5. Serve immediately and enjoy!

Each serving contains 362 Calories, 27.4g Fats, 3.2g Net Carbs, and 22.3g Protein.

FRESH BACON AND CHICKEN PATTIES

Ingredients

- 1 (12 oz.) Can Chicken Breast
- 1 Large Egg
- 4 Slices Bacon
- 2 Medium Bell Peppers
- 1/4 Cup Sun Dried Tomato Pesto
- 1/4 Cup Parmesan Cheese
- 3 Tbsp. Coconut Flour

Directions

1. Fry the bacon until crisp on both sides.

2. In a food processor, chop 2 bell peppers and then scoop mixture into a bowl. Pat any excess moisture out with paper towels.

3. Chop chicken and bacon together in food processor until smooth. Add to pepper mixture. Add parmesan, coconut flour, eggs and tomato pesto into the mixture and mix everything together.

4. Form the patties and fry on medium-high heat in a pan. Once browned, flip over, continue cooking, and remove to paper towels when finished.

5. Serve immediately and enjoy!

Each servings contains 159 Calories, 11.5g Fats, 1.7g Net Carbs, and 9.9g Protein.

KETO ASIAN GRILLED SHORT RIBS

Ingredients

Ribs and Marinade

- 6 large Short Ribs
- 1/4 cup Soy Sauce
- 2 tbsp. Fish Sauce
- 2 tbsp. Rice Vinegar

Asian Spice Rub

- 1 tsp. Ground Ginger
- 1/2 tsp. Onion Powder
- 1/2 tsp, Minced Garlic
- 1/2 tsp. Red Pepper Flakes
- 1/2 tsp. Sesame Seed
- 1/4 tsp. Cardamom
- 1 tbsp. Salt

Directions

1. Mix the marinade together and marinate ribs for 1 hour. Mix together the spice rub and evenly coat the ribs with the rub.

2. Grill the ribs for 3-5 minutes per side.

3. Serve immediately and enjoy!

Each serving contains 417 Calories, 31.8g Fats, 0.9g Net Carbs, and 29.5g Protein.

CHEESY BACON CHEESEBURGER

Ingredients

- 2 Slices Bacon, pre-cooked
- 8 oz. Ground Beef
- 2 oz. Cheddar Cheese
- 1 oz. Mozzarella Cheese
- 1 tbsp. Butter
- 1 tsp. Cajun Seasoning
- 1 tsp. Salt
- 1/2 tsp. Pepper

Directions

1. Season ground beef with spices and make patties stuffed with mozzarella. For each burger, heat 1 tbsp. butter in a pan. Add the burger to the pan and cover.

2. Cook for 3 minutes, cover with cloche, and continue cooking until desired results. Chop the bacon slices in half and place over the top of the burgers.

3. Serve immediately and enjoy!

Each burger contains 614 Calories, 51g Fats, 1.5g Net Carbs, and 33g Protein.

KETO SESAME BEEF

Ingredients

- 1 lb. Rib eye Steak, sliced into ¼" strips
- 1 medium Daikon Radish
- ½ medium Red Pepper, sliced into thin strips
- ½ medium Jalapeno Pepper, sliced into thin rings
- 1 medium Green Onion, chopped
- 1 clove Garlic, minced
- 4 tbsp. Soy Sauce 1 tbsp. Coconut Oil
- 1 tbsp. + 1 tsp. Rice Vinegar
- 1 tbsp. Toasted Sesame Seeds
- 1 tbsp. Coconut Flour
- 1 tsp. Ginger, minced
- 1 tsp. Sesame Oil
- 1 tsp. Sriracha or Sambal Olek
- 1 tsp. Oyster Sauce
- 1/2 tsp. Guar Gum
- ½ tsp. Red Pepper Flakes
- 7 drops Liquid Stevia
- Coconut Oil for frying

Directions

1. Use a spiralizer, slice the daikon radish into noodle-like strings. Soak the daikon noodles in a bowl of cold water for 20 minutes.

2. Chop the rib eye steak into small strips. Coat with coconut flour and guar gum. Let marinate for 10 minutes. Prepare the vegetables.

3. Heat oil in a wok. Add the garlic, ginger, and red pepper. Fry for 2 minutes until aromatic. Add the soy sauce, oyster sauce, sesame oil, rice vinegar, stevia and sriracha. Whisk together and cook for 1-2 minutes longer.

4. Heat oil in a large pot until it reaches 325 F. Add the beef strips and fry for 2-3 minutes on each side. Remove the beef from the oil and place on paper towels to absorb some of the oil. Combine the beef with the vegetables and stir together with sauce. Cook for another 2 minutes.

5. Drain the daikon radish noodles and divide them onto each serving plate. Top each with sesame beef.

6. Serve immediately and enjoy!

Each serving contains 412 calories, 31.3g Fats, 5g Net Carbs, and 24.5g Protein.

BEEF WRAPS WITH SALSA

Ingredients

- 32 small sardines – rinsed
- 8 tbsp. extra-virgin olive oil
- 4 tbsp. freshly chopped mint
- 4 tbsp. basil
- Salt and pepper, to taste

Directions

1. Preheat oven to 350 F.

2. Prepare vegetables according to directions. Add the lard in a large skillet over medium heat. Stir in the onions and garlic.

3. Place sardines on a rack and season with salt and pepper. Bake in the oven for 10 minutes. Once cooked, top with fresh herbs and olive oil.

4. Serve immediately and enjoy!

Each serving contains 482 calories, 40g Fats, 0.41g Net Carbs, and 40.1g Protein.

TARTE TATIN

Ingredients:

- 1 1/2 cup almond flour
- 1 cup grated parmesan cheese
- 1/2 cup basil pesto
- 1/3 cup flax meal
- 1 large egg
- 2 lb. tomatoes
- 1 package mozzarella cheese
- 1 tbsp. freshly chopped oregano
- 3 tbsp. butter or ghee
- 2 tbsp. fresh basil
- 1 tsp dried oregano
- 1 tsp dried basil
- Salt and pepper, to taste.

Directions:

1. Preheat oven to 400 F.

2. Combine the dry ingredients into a mixing bowl. Grate the parmesan cheese. Add the melted butter and eggs. Place the mixture onto a non-stick pan and bake for 10 minutes.

3. Remove from heat and add the tomatoes. Top with basil pesto and mozzarella and return to the oven. Bake for another 20 minutes.

4. Serve immediately and enjoy!

Each serving contains 425 calories, 36g Fats, 11.8g Net Carbs, and 16.1g Protein.

KETOGENIC FOR VEGETARIAN

VEGETARIAN BREAKFAST

Ingredients

- 1 large egg – fried
- ½ avocado
- 1 oz. cheddar cheese
- 1 cup mushrooms
- ⅓ Cup sauerkraut
- ½ cup cooked spinach
- 2 tbsp. ghee
- Salt and pepper, to taste.

Directions

1. Cook the mushrooms and spinach in 1 tbsp. ghee. Add the remaining ghee to the egg and season with salt and pepper.

2. Serve with cheese, sauerkraut, and avocado.

3. Enjoy!

Each serving contains 623 Calories, 55.5g Fats, 6.7g Net Carbs, and 19.8g Protein.

KETO MIXED GREEN SALAD

Ingredients

- 2 slices Bacon
- 2 oz. Mixed Greens
- 3 tbsp. Pine Nuts, roasted
- 2 tbsp. Shaved Parmesan
- 2 tbsp. Keto Raspberry Vinaigrette (see condiments)
- Salt and Pepper, to taste

Directions

1. Cook bacon in a pan until nice and crisp. Crumble the bacon and add to mixed salad along with the rest of the ingredients. Mix salad until well dressed.

2. Serve immediately and enjoy!

Each serving contains 478 Calories, 37g Fats, 4g Net Carbs, and 17g Protein.

BOK CHOY AND TOFU SALAD

Ingredients

Baked Tofu

- 15 oz. Extra Firm Tofu
- 1/2 Lemon – juiced
- 1 tbsp. Rice Wine Vinegar
- 1 tbsp. Sesame Oil
- 1 tbsp. Soy Sauce
- 1 tbsp. Water
- 2 tsp. Minced Garlic

Boy Choy Salad

- 9 oz. Bok Choy
- 1 stalk Green Onion
- 3 tbsp. Coconut Oil
- 2 tbsp. Soy Sauce
- 2 tbsp. Cilantro, chopped
- 1 tbsp. Sambal Olek
- 1 tbsp. Peanut Butter
- 1/2 lime – juice
- 7 drops Liquid Stevia

Directions

1. Pre-heat oven to 350 F.

2. Allow the tofu to dry for about 5-6 hours. Combine sesame oil, soy sauce, garlic, vinegar, water, and lemon for the marinade. Cut the tofu into squares and place in a plastic bag mixed with the marinade. Allow to marinate for at least 30 minutes, preferably overnight.

3. Place tofu on a baking sheet lined with parchment paper and bake for 30 minutes. Mix the salad dressing ingredients together in a bowl, except the bok choy. Add cilantro and spring onion.

4. Slice the Bok choy into small portions. Remove the tofu from heat. Arrange your salad to proper proportions.

5. Serve immediately and enjoy!

Each serving contains 442.3 Calories, 35g Fats, 5.6g Net Carbs, and 25g Protein.

KETO CAPRESE SALAD

Ingredients

- 6 Oz. Fresh Mozzarella Cheese
- 1 Tomato
- 1/4 Cup Fresh Basil, chopped
- 3 tbsp. Olive Oil
- Salt and pepper, to taste

Directions

1. In a food processor, pulse the chopped fresh basil leaves with 2 tbsp. Olive Oil to make the Basil Paste.

2. Slice the tomato into 1/4" slices. Cut the Mozzarella into 1 oz. Slices.

3. Assemble the Caprese salad by layering tomato, mozzarella, and the basil paste. Season with salt, pepper, and extra olive oil.

4. Serve immediately and enjoy!

Each serving contains 405 Calories, 36g Fats, 4.5g Net Carbs, and 15.5g Protein.

RED COCONUT CURRY

Ingredients

Coconut Curry Chicken

- 5 Chicken Thighs, deboned with skin
- 1 large Egg
- 1/2 cup Unsweetened Shredded Coconut
- 1/2 cup Pork Rinds, crumbled
- 2 tsp. Curry Powder
- 1/2 tsp. Coriander
- 1/4 tsp. Onion Powder
- 1/4 tsp. Garlic Powder
- Salt and Pepper, to Taste

Sweet and Spicy Mango Sauce

- 1/4 cup Sour Cream
- 1/4 cup Mayonnaise
- 2 tbsp. Sugar Free Ketchup
- 1 1/2 tsp. Mango Extract
- 1/2 tsp. Ground Ginger
- 1/2 tsp. Red Pepper Flakes
- 1/2 tsp. Garlic Powder
- 1/4 tsp. Cayenne Pepper
- 7 drops Liquid Stevia

Directions

1. Pre-heat oven to 400 F.

2. In a shallow bowl, beat the egg. Remove bones from the chicken thighs with skin on, then cut chicken into strips or cubes.

3. In large plastic bag, place the pork rinds, spices, and coconut. Add the chicken and shake until well combined. Place the tenders on the wire rack and bake for 15 minutes. Flip the chicken and bake for another 20 minutes.

4. Combine all the sauce ingredients and mix together. Serve with chicken tenders.

5. Enjoy!

Each serving contains 494 Calories, 39.4g Fats, 2.1g Net Carbs, and 29.4g Protein.

LOW-CARB MUSHROOM CAULIFLOWER RISOTTO

Ingredients

- 4 medium Baby Bella Mushrooms
- 2 cups Cauliflower, riced
- 1 cup Chicken Broth
- 1/4 cup Parmesan Cheese
- 1/4 cup Heavy Cream
- 2 cloves Garlic
- 1 tbsp. Olive Oil
- 1 tsp. Tarragon
- Salt and Pepper, to taste

Directions

1. Chop cauliflower florets and place in a food processor. Blend until rice sized.

2. In a pan, cook the garlic and mushrooms in olive oil over medium heat. Once the garlic is fragrant, add the chicken broth and cauliflower. Stirring constantly.

3. Reduce heat to a simmer and cover. Let steam for 5-7 minutes.

4. When the cauliflower is cooked, remove the cover and let the chicken broth evaporate for about 5-10 minutes. Once the moisture is evaporated, add the parmesan cheese, heavy cream and spices. Stir until parmesan has melted.

5. Serve immediately and enjoy!

Each serving contains 246 Calories, 19.9g Fats, 6.0g Net Carbs, and 7g Protein.

KETO CREAMY SPINACH

Ingredients

- 10 oz. Frozen Spinach
- 3 oz. Cream Cheese
- 3 tbsp. Parmesan Cheese
- 2 tbsp. Sour Cream
- 1/4 tsp. Onion Powder
- 1/4 tsp. Garlic Powder
- Salt and Pepper, to Taste

Directions

1. Allow the frozen spinach to defrost. Place the spinach in the pan over medium-high heat. Add the cream cheese and seasoning to the pan. Stir constantly until cream cheese has melted.

2. Add the sour cream and parmesan and mix together well until the creamed spinach is thick.

3. Serve immediately and enjoy!

Each serving contains 157. Calories, 13.2g Fats, 2g Net Carbs, and 5.6g Protein.

EGG SALAD STUFFED AVOCADO

Ingredients

- 6 large Hard Boiled Eggs
- 3 medium Avocados
- 3 stalks Celery
- 1/3 medium Red Onion
- 4 tbsp. Mayonnaise
- 2 tbsp. Fresh Lime Juice
- 2 tsp. Brown Mustard
- 1 tsp. Hot Sauce
- 1/2 tsp. Cumin
- Salt and Pepper, to taste

Directions

1. Prep all ingredients by chopping eggs, celery, and onions. Combine the ingredients in a bowl except for avocado. Slice the avocados in half and remove the pits. Spoon 2-3 tbsp. of egg salad into each avocado.

2. Serve immediately and enjoy!

Each serving contains 299 Calories, 27.3g Fats, 3.8g Net Carbs, and 8.2g Protein.

AUTHENTIC GREEK SALAD

Ingredients

- 16 Kalamata olives
- 1 large cucumber - sliced
- 1 medium green pepper – halved, deseed
- 1 small red onion - sliced
- 4-5 medium tomatoes – sliced
- 1 cup feta cheese
- 4 tbsp. capers
- 4 tbsp. extra virgin olive oil
- 1 tsp oregano, dried
- Salt and pepper, to taste

Directions

1. Prepare vegetables according to directions. Place into a bowl and add the capers, oregano, and olives. Add the feta cheese and drizzle with olive oil.

2. Serve immediately and enjoy!

Each serving contains 323 Calories, 27.8 Fats, 8g Net Carbs, and 9.3g Protein.

KETO VEGETABLE LASAGNA

Ingredients

- 300 g fresh spinach
- 2 medium eggplants
- 6 large eggs
- 1 cup Marinara sauce
- 1 cup mozzarella cheese, grated
- 1 ⅓ cup feta cheese - crumbled
- ½ cup parmesan cheese, grated
- ¼ cup + 2 tbsp. ghee
- ½ tsp Salt

Directions

1. Preheat oven to 400 F.

2. Slice the eggplant into ½ inch cuts and place on a baking tray. With the eggplants with melted ghee and season with salt. Bake for 20 minutes.

3. Blanch the fresh spinach by bringing a pot to a boil over high heat. Fill another bowl with ice cold water. Place the spinach into the boiled water for 30-60 seconds then immediately transfer the leaves onto the iced water. Remove cooled, remove from the cold water and drain.

4. Once the eggplant is done, remove from heat and set aside. Reduce the oven temp. to 360 F.

5. Prepare the omelets by cracking one egg at a time and season with salt. Mix well. Pour the egg mixture in a hot pan greased with ghee and swirl until you achieve a thin omelet – cook for 1 minute. Place on a plate and repeat – making a total of 5-6 omelets.

6. Heat the marinara sauce and assemble the lasagna by layering 2 omelets on the bottom of the dish. Spread the marina sauce and add another layer of eggplant slices. Top with mozzarella and spinach.

7. Add another layer of two more omelets with feta cheese. Repeat the laying process in the order of marinara sauce, eggplant slices, mozzarella, spinach, and feta cheese.

8. For the final layer, add the remaining omelets and ingredients. Top with parmesan cheese and place in the oven. Bake for 25 minutes, until golden brown.

9. Remove from heat and let cool.

10. Serve immediately and enjoy!

Each serving contains 474 Calories, 38 Fats, 8.7g Net Carbs, and 20.8g Protein.

KETO VEGETARIAN BURGER

Ingredients

Marinated & grilled mushrooms

- 2 medium large flat mushrooms such as Portobello
- 1 clove garlic, crushed
- 1 tbsp. coconut oil
- 1 tbsp. freshly chopped oregano
- 1/2 tbsp. freshly chopped basil
- ¼ tsp salt
- Ground black pepper

Toppings

- 2 Keto buns
- 2 large eggs
- 2 slices cheddar cheese
- 1 cup mixed lettuce
- 2 tbsp. Keto mayo

Directions

1. Toast the Keto buns and prepare the mushrooms. Season with salt and pepper then add fresh herbs, coconut oil, crushed garlic. Marinate for 1 hour.

2. Cook the mushrooms on a hot pan over medium-high heat. Flip on the other side for another 5 minutes. Remove from heat and top each with cheese slices.

3. Fry the eggs in ghee and use molds to create shapes for the burger. Assemble the burgers by adding mayo on each Keto bun halves. Add the mushrooms, eggs, tomato, and lettuce.

4. Serve immediately and enjoy!

Each serving contains 637 Calories, 55.1 Fats, 8.7g Net Carbs, and 23.7g Protein.

KETO ASIAN CUCUMBER SALAD

Ingredients

- 1 packet Shirataki Noodles
- 3/4 large Cucumber
- 1 medium Spring Onion
- 2 tbsp. Coconut Oil
- 1 tbsp. Sesame Oil
- 1 tbsp. Rice Vinegar
- 1/4 tsp. Red Pepper Flakes
- 1 tsp. Sesame Seeds
- Salt and Pepper, to Taste

Directions

1. Rinse off the shirataki noodles. Make sure you get the excess water and wash them off completely. Set them on a paper towel to dry.

2. Bring 2 tbsp. Coconut Oil to medium-high temperature in a pan. Once pan is hot, fry the noodles for 5-7 minutes. Remove from pan and set aside on a paper towel to cool.

3. Thinly slice the cucumber, then arrange on a plate. Add the rest of the ingredients over the cucumber and let the dish chill in the fridge for at least 30 minutes. Sprinkle the fried shiitake noodles over the top!

4. Serve immediately and enjoy!

Each serving contains 416 Calories, 43g Fats, 7g Net Carbs, and 2g Protein.

LOW-CARB FALAFEL

Ingredients

- 1 cup chickpeas
- 1 cup riced cauliflower
- 1/3 cup frozen peas and carrots
- 1/4 cup tahini
- 1/4 cup diced red onion
- 1/4 cup lemon juice
- 1 tbsp. dried parsley
- 2 tsp cumin
- 1 tsp garlic powder
- 1 tsp salt
- 1/4 tsp all spice

Directions

1. Preheat oven to 350 F. Line a cookie sheet with parchment paper.

2. Add the ingredients to a high speed blender and blend for 30 seconds until well combined. Blend for another 15-30 seconds, until paste results.

3. Remove the ingredients from the blender and scoop the "dough" into 14 equal portions on the tray, about 1/2 inch thick. Bake for 25 minutes. Let cool.

4. Serve immediately and enjoy!

Each serving contains 50 Calories, 2.8g Fats, 3g Net Carbs, and 1.7g Protein.

KETO GNOCCHI

Ingredients

- 2 cups Mozzarella
- 3 eggs – separated yolk
- 1 tsp garlic
- Extra-virgin olive oil
- Butter

Directions

1. Place the garlic and cheese in a microwave safe bowl and mix well to combine. Melt cheese in microwave for about 1 to 1 1/2 minutes. Fold in one egg yolk at a time, Portion the dough into four balls.

2. Allow to chill for least 10 minutes. Lightly grease the parchment and roll out each ball into a 14″ log. Slice each log into one-inch pieces.

3. In a large pot, bring about a 1/2 gallon of salted water to a boil. Place the gnocchi into the pot and cook until they float, about 2-3 minutes. Strain the gnocchi.

4. Heat the large pan over medium-high heat. Add a butter and a tablespoon of oil to pan. Stir in the gnocchi and sauté each side for about 1-2 minutes, until golden. Season with salt and pepper.

5. Serve immediately and enjoy!

Each serving contains 324 Calories, 27g Fats, 3g Net Carbs, and 18g Protein.

KETO VEGETARIAN ZOODLES

Ingredients

- 4 medium zucchini sliced using a spiralizer
- 2 avocados
- 1 cup Kalamata olives, pitted
- ½ cup Paleo Avocado Pesto
- ¼ cup fresh basil
- ¼ cup sun-dried tomatoes, drained, 4-6 halves
- 2 tbsp. extra virgin coconut oil
- ¼ tsp salt or more to taste

Directions

1. Prepare the zucchini noodles using a spiralizer. Place the "zoodles" in a pan with coconut oil and cook for 3 minutes. Halve the avocado and remove the seeds, cut into stripes. Drain the tomatoes and olives.

2. Remove the zoodles from heat and add the pesto sauce. Season with salt and mix until combined. Place the ingredients on a serve plate and enjoy!

Each serving contains 449 Calories, 41.7g Fats, 8.4g Net Carbs, and 6.3g Protein.

KETO STUFFED EGGPLANT

Ingredients

- 6 eggplants
- 4 garlic cloves, minced
- 4 tomatoes, chopped
- 2 medium red onions, chopped
- 1 green bell pepper, seeded and chopped
- 4 tbsp. olive oil
- 3 tbsp. chopped fresh parsley
- 1 tsp. raw coconut palm sugar
- 1 tsp. ground cumin
- 1 tbsp. tomato paste
- Salt and pepper, to taste

Directions

1. Preheat the oven to 450 F.

2. Place a rack in the middle lined with a baking sheet and brush with olive oil. Using a vegetable peeler, remove the skin of the eggplant.

3. Cut the eggplants open lengthwise. Sprinkle salt on each eggplant, then set them all in a colander and rest for about 1 hour. Place on the baking sheet and bake for 20 minutes. Remove heat and set aside.

4. In the meantime, heat olive oil over medium heat in a large skillet and add the onions, stirring occasionally. Add the bell pepper and garlic. Continue to cook until the vegetables are tender - about 10 minutes. Season with salt and pepper, then stir in the chopped tomato, cumin,

sugar, parsley and tomato paste. Cook for another 5 minutes, until fragrant. Set aside.

5. Reduce heat to 350 F.

6. Arrange the eggplants in the baking dish so that each one is butterflied open. Season with salt and fill with the onion mixture. Drizzle with remaining olive oil, add two tablespoons of water to the baking dish and bake for about 40 to 45 minutes.

7. The eggplants should be flat and the liquid in the pan slightly caramelized.

8. Serve immediately and enjoy!

Each serving contains 116 calories, 12g fat, 11g carbs, and 3g protein.

KETO VEGGIE TIKKA MASALA

Ingredients

- 3 cans chickpeas, drained and rinsed
- 2 cans diced tomatoes
- 1 can full fat coconut milk
- 1 large onion, finely chopped
- 2 garlic cloves, minced
- 1 2-inch piece of ginger, finely chopped
- 2 tbsp. olive oil
- 2 tsp. ground cumin
- 2 tsp. ground coriander
- 2 tsp. paprika
- 1 tsp. arrowroot powder
- 1 tsp. Garam Masala
- 1 tsp. turmeric
- ½ tsp. cayenne pepper
- Salt, to taste

Directions

1. Add olive oil in a large saucepan over medium-high heat. Add the onions and salt, then sauté until translucent, about 6 minutes, stirring frequently.

2. Add the garlic and stir for another minute. Add the ginger and spices.

3. Add the diced tomatoes and chickpeas. Bring the mixture to a boil. Reduce heat to a low simmer for another 15 minutes. Pour the coconut milk. Simmer for 5 minutes.

4. In a small bowl whisk the arrowroot powder with 2 tablespoons of water. Stir in the chickpea mixture and cook for another 5 minutes, until the gravy has thickened. Remove from heat top and with chopped fresh cilantro.

5. Serve immediately and enjoy!

Each serving contains 393 calories, 13g fat, 60g carbs, and 15g protein

SPICED BROCCOLI

Ingredients

- 2 small broccoli
- 2 tsp freshly chopped chili pepper
- 2 tbsp. contemporary ginger
- 4 cloves garlic
- Juice from 2 limes
- 8 tbsp. sesame oil

Directions

1. Prepare the broccoli and break into florets. Place the broccoli in a steamer.

2. Meanwhile, grate the ginger root and garlic. Chop the chili pepper and halve the lime. Squeeze the lime juice into a bowl. Add balsamic vinegar, sesame oil, and the rest of the ingredients.

3. Place the broccoli onto a plate and pour the dressing.

4. Serve immediately and enjoy!

Each serving contains 294 calories, 26.6g fat, 13.9g carbs, and 4.6g protein.

AVOCADO AND KALE SALAD

Ingredients

- 1 medium avocado
- 2 cups chopped kale
- 1/2 lime - juiced
- 1/2 orange – juiced
- 2 tbsp. hazelnut oil
- 2 tbsp. pine nuts
- 1/2 tsp sea salt and black pepper

Directions

1. Add 2 liters of water into a pot and bring to a boil. Add salt. Wash the kale ad add to the bot. Remove the kale and let it cool.

2. Chop the kale into small pieces and place in a serving bowl. Remove the skins of the avocado and cut into cubes. Prepare the dressing by combining the juices, hazelnut oil, and pepper. Mix well. Add the avocado into the bowl and pour the dressing

3. Serve immediately and enjoy!

Each serving contains 379 calories, 34.9g fat, 18g carbs, and 5.3g protein.

KETO POTATO SALAD

Ingredients

- 1⁄2 medium cauliflower
- 1⁄2 medium celery root
- 8 crispy bacon slices
- 2 eggs
- 2 carrots
- 1 parsley root
- 1⁄2 cup diced pickled cucumbers
- 4 tbsp. bitter cream
- 2 tbsp. parsley
- 2 tbsp. mayonnaise
- 1 tbsp. contemporary dill
- Salt and black pepper, to taste

Directions

1. Peel the parsley, celery root and carrot. Cut the cauliflower into quarter size and place into a pot with salt and water. Bring to a boil.

2. Meanwhile, boil the eggs. Once cooked, allow to chill over cold water then peel the shell.

3. Slice the parsley, celery and carrot into small cuts. Add the shallot into a bowl. Cut the cucumber into cubes and add the eggs into the bowl with the greens.

4. Combine the mayonnaise and bitter cream in a separate bowl and mix.

5. Mix the ingredients and add the chopped parsley and dill. Add the mayo mixture and season with salt and pepper.

6. Serve immediately and enjoy!

Each serving contains 380 calories, 25.9g fat, 19.4g carbs, and 21.8g protein.

SIDE & SNACKS RECIPES

KETO CORNDOG MUFFINS

Ingredients

- 1 large Egg
- 1/2 cup Almond Flour
- 1/2 cup Flaxseed Meal
- 1/3 cup Sour Cream
- 1/4 cup Butter, melted
- 1/4 cup Coconut Milk
- 3 tbsp. Swerve Sweetener
- 1 tbsp. Psyllium Husk Powder
- 1/4 tsp. Baking Powder
- 3 hot dogs
- Salt

Directions

1. Pre-heat oven to 375 F.

2. Mix the dry ingredients in a bowl. Add the egg, coconut milk, sour cream and butter and mix well.

3. Divide the batter into muffin slots. Slice the hot dogs in thirds and insert into the middle of each muffin tin.

4. Bake for 12 minutes. Then broil for 2 minutes until tops are browned. Allow the muffins cool.

Each serving contains 80 calories, 6.9g fat, 0.6g carbs, and 2.5g protein.

KETO CASHEW NUTTY BARS

Ingredients

- 1 cup Almond Flour
- 1/2 cup Cashews
- 1/4 cup Keto Maple Syrup
- 1/4 cup Shredded Coconut
- 1/4 cup Butter - melted
- 1 tsp. Cinnamon
- 1 pinch Salt

Directions

1. Combine almond flour and butter in a bowl and combine. Add the shredded coconut, maple syrup, cinnamon, and salt. Mix well.

2. Chop 1/2 cup of cashews and add to the dough.

3. Line baking sheet with parchment paper and spread dough evenly. Place the bar in the refrigerator and chill for 3 hours.

4. Serve and enjoy!

Each serving contains 190 calories, 18g fat, 4g carbs, and 4g protein.

LOW-CARB CHIA BARS

Ingredients

- 3 oz. Shredded Cheddar Cheese
- 1 cup Ice Water
- 1/2 cup Chia Seeds
- 2 tbsps. Olive Oil
- 2 tbsps. Psyllium Husk Powder
- 1/4 tsp. Xanthan Gum
- 1/4 tsp. Onion Powder
- 1/4 tsp. Garlic Powder
- 1/4 tsp. Paprika
- 1/4 tsp. Oregano
- Salt and Pepper

Directions

1. Preheat your oven to 375F.

2. Grind chia seeds. Add the dry ingredients and ground chia seeds into a bowl. Add the olive oil and combine with the dry ingredients.

3. Pour water into bowl and mix until you form the dough. Add the shredded cheddar mix the cheese into the dough. Set onto a baking sheet and let sit. Spread the dough thinly over the baking sheet.

4. Bake for 30 minutes.

5. Remove from heat and cut into individual pieces. Return the chia bars into the oven and broil for 5 minutes or until crackers are crisped.

6. Serve immediately and enjoy!

Each serving contains 30 calories, 2.5g fat, 0g carbs, and 1.3g protein.

KETO CHOCOLATE COOKIES

Ingredients

- 1 Egg
- 5 bars 95%+ Cocoa Bar
- 1 cup Almond Flour
- 1/4 cup Erythritol
- 3 tbsps. Whey Protein
- 2 tbsps. Psyllium Husk
- 2 tbsps. Coconut Flour
- 8 tbsps. Butter
- 2 tsps. Vanilla Extract
- 1/2 tsp. Baking Powder
- 10 drops Liquid Stevia

Directions

1. Preheat oven to 350F.

2. Mix the dry ingredient together. Add the erythritol and stevia. Add the egg and vanilla extract. Mix together until well-combined. Sift together. Chop the cocoa into chunks and mix into the dough.

3. Roll dough and scoop 18 balls. Place on a baking sheet and flatten the balls to form a cookie. Bake for 15 minutes, or until golden.

4. Serve immediately and enjoy!

Each serving contains 120 calories, 11g fat, 1.5g carbs, and 2.5g protein.

BACON CHEESE BOMBS

Ingredients

- 10 slices Bacon
- 8 oz. Mozzarella Cheese
- 1 Egg
- 4 tbsps. Butter - melted
- 4 tbsps. Almond Flour
- 3 tbsps. Psyllium Husk Powder
- 1/3 tsp. Garlic Powder
- 1/3 tsp. Onion Powder
- 1 cup Oil
- Salt and Black pepper

Directions

1. Microwave half of the cheese until gooey. Microwave butter until fully melted, then pour butter into egg and cheese.

2. Add the almond flour, Psyllium husk and spices. Mix until well combined. Pour the dough onto a sheet. Roll dough into a large rectangle. Fill rectangle with rest of cheese and cover completely. Cut into 20 squares.

3. Tightly wrap each piece in bacon, using toothpicks to secure the bacon.

4. Heat oil to 350 degrees, then fry for 3 minutes each until golden and crisp. Remove from oil and let cool on paper towels to drain.

5. Serve immediately and enjoy!

Each serving contains 90 calories, 7g fat, 0.6g carbs, and 6g protein.

EGGPLANT FRIES

Ingredients

- 4 eggplants
- 2 cups parmesan cheese - grated
- 1 cup flaxseed
- 4 tsp basil
- 4 tsp oregano (dried)
- 4 eggs
- 8 tbsp. marinara sauce

Directions

1. Preheat oven to 400 F.

2. Pour the flaxseed in a processor and pulse until powdered results. Add the grated parmesan cheese and mix with the flax meal and herbs.

3. Beat the eggs and add salt. Cut the eggplant into fries. Dip the eggplant fries into egg, then the herb and flax mixture and repeat on the egg.

4. Place the eggplant fries on a cooking tray with parchment paper and spray with cooking oil. Bake for 15-20 minutes or until golden.

5. Serve immediately with marinara sauce and enjoy!

Each serving contains 456 calories, 29 g fat, 8g carbs, and 27g protein.

KETO FLAX TORTILLAS

Ingredients

- 1 cup + 2 tbsp. Water
- 1 cup Golden Flax Seed Meal
- 2 tbsps. Psyllium Husk Powder
- 2 tsps. Olive Oil
- 1/2 tsp. Curry Powder
- 1/4 tsp. Xanthan Gum
- Coconut Flour
- Extra Olive Oil

Directions

1. Mix all the dry ingredients together, then add the water and 2 tsp. oil. Mix until the dough forms. Let sit for 1 hour, uncovered.

2. Split the tortilla into 3 portions if you are rolling by hand. Press your hand down and sprinkle coconut flour over the face of the tortilla and roll until thin.

3. Heat oil in a pan over medium-high heat and fry until desired.

Each serving contains 165 calories, 19.3 g fat, 0.5g carbs, and 6.5g protein.

KETO TORTILLA CHIPS

Ingredients

- 6 Flaxseed Tortillas (recipe above)
- 3 tbsps. Olive Oil
- Salt and Pepper, to Taste

Directions

1. Prepare the Tortillas according to recipe. Preheat the deep fryer.

2. Cut the tortillas into 6 or 8 slices. Once ready, place 4-6 pieces at a time and fry for 1-2 minutes each. Flip and fry for another minute.

3. Remove from oil and place on a paper towel to cool. Season with salt and pepper, to taste.

4. Serve with your favorite toppings of choice.

Each 12 servings contain 9 calories, 1g fat, 0g carbs, and 0.3g protein.

KETO CHEESEBURGER MUFFIN

Ingredients

Cheeseburger Muffin Buns

- 2 large Eggs
- 1/2 cup Almond Flour
- 1/2 cup Flaxseed Meal
- 1/4 cup Sour Cream
- 1 tsp. Baking Powder
- Salt and pepper

Hamburger Filling

- 16 oz. Ground Beef
- 2 tbsps. Tomato Paste
- 1/2 tsp. Garlic Powder
- 1/2 tsp. Onion Powder
- Salt and Pepper to Taste

Toppings

- 18 slices Dill Pickles
- 1/2 cup Cheddar Cheese
- 2 tbsps. Mustard
- 2 tbsps. Keto Ketchup

Directions

1. Cook the ground beef in a hot pan with seasonings.

2. Mix the dry ingredients together and pre-heat oven to 350 F. Stir in the wet ingredients.

3. Pour the mixture into silicone muffin cups. Make an indent on the muffin for the ground beef. Fill each muffin with the beef mixture.

4. Bake for 20 minutes, until muffins are golden on the outside. Remove from heat and top with cheese, then broil for another 3 minutes. Allow to cool for 5 minutes, and then remove from the silicone muffin cups.

5. Serve and enjoy!

Each serving contains 245calories, 18g fat, 2g carbs, and 14.1g protein.

CHIA ALMOND BUTTER BARS

Ingredients

- 1/2 cup Coconut Cream
- 1/2 cup Unsweetened Shredded Coconut Flakes
- 1/2 cup Almonds
- 1/4 cup Heavy Cream
- 1/4 cup Chia Seeds
- 4 tbsps. Erythritol
- 2 tbsps. Coconut Flour
- 2 tbsps. Butter
- 1 1/2 tsp. Vanilla Extract
- 1 tbsp. + 1 tsp. Coconut Oil
- 1/4 tsp. Liquid Stevia

Directions

1. Grind toasted almonds in food processor. Add 2 tbsp. erythritol and 1 tsp. coconut oil and mix until almond butter is formed.

2. Heat butter in a pan. Add heavy cream, 2 tbsp. erythritol, stevia, and vanilla. Mix until bubbly. Add the almond butter and stir.

3. While the almond butter mixture is cooking, grind the chia seeds. Mix the chia seeds and coconut flakes in a pan to toast for 1 minute.

4. Add the coconut cream, coconut flour, 1 tbsp. coconut oil. Mix until well-combined.

5. Chill for 1 hour. Chop into small squares and serve.

Each serving contains 120 calories, 11g fat, 1.3g carbs, and 2.3g protein.

SESAME LEMON CUMIN MUG CAKE

Ingredients

Base

- 1 Egg
- 2 Tbsp. Almond Flour
- 2 Tbsp. Butter
- 1/2 tsp. Baking Powder

Flavor

- 1 Tbsp. Sesame Seed
- 1 tsp. Lemon Juice
- 1/4 tsp. Pepper
- 1/4 tsp. Cumin
- Salt

Directions

1. Combine the ingredients together and mix. Place in the microwave and 60-75 seconds on high. Remove the cake from the mug and add lemon zest to top.

2. Serve immediately and enjoy!

Each serving contains 410 calories, 36g fat, 3g carbs, and 11g protein.

SPINACH LATTE

Ingredients

- 1 Cup Coffee
- 3/4 Cup Coconut Milk
- 1/2 Cup Pumpkin Puree
- 2 Handfuls Spinach
- 2 Tbsp. Erythritol
- 2 Tbsp. Butter
- 1/2 tsp. Cinnamon
- 1/2 tsp. Vanilla Extract
- 1/4 tsp. Allspice
- 1/4 tsp. Ginger
- 1/4 tsp. Cardamom
- 10 drops Liquid Stevia
- 2 Handfuls of Ice

Directions

1. Combine ingredients together in a blender. Top with cinnamon and whipped cream.

2. Serve immediately and enjoy!

Each serving contains 154 calories, 13g fat, 3g carbs, and 2.3g protein.

SALTED CARAMEL PORK RINDS

Ingredients

- 1 oz. Pork Rinds
- 1 Cup Unsweetened Vanilla Coconut Milk
- 2 Tbsp. Heavy Cream
- 2 Tbsp. Butter
- 1 Tbsp. Erythritol
- 1/4 tsp. Ground Cinnamon

Directions

1. Add 2 Tbsp. Butter to pan over medium heat. Remove from heat and add erythritol and heavy cream. Mix well and return heat.

2. Allow the caramel mixture to bubble. Mix well.

3. Once the caramel is well cooked, add pork rinds and mix them in. Make sure that the pork rinds are coated.

4. Transfer pork rinds to a container and place in the fridge for 30 minutes.

5. Serve with milk and enjoy!

Each serving contains 510 calories, 46g fat, 2.6g carbs, and 14g protein.

PAN-FRIED QUESO FRESCO

Ingredients

- 1 package Queso Fresco
- 1 Tbsp. Extra-virgin Coconut Oil
- 1/2 Tbsp. Olive Oil

Directions

1. Cut cheese into thin rectangles.

2. Add Coconut Oil and Olive Oil to a pan over high heat. Once you reach the smoking point, add the cheese.

3. Cook until browned on one side and then flip over and continue until browned.

4. Remove from heat and drain on a paper towel.

5. Serve immediately and enjoy!

Each serving contains 240 calories, 19g fat, 0g carbs, and 16g protein.

GLAZED SPICED LEMON FRITTERS

Ingredients

Spice Fritters

- 1 Large Egg 1/2 Cup Almond Flour
- 2 Cups olive oil
- 3 Tbsp. Erythritol
- 1 tsp. Baking Powder
- 1/2 tsp. Cinnamon
- 1/2 tsp. Xanthan Gum
- 1/2 tsp. Vanilla
- Zest of 1/2 Lemon

Lemon Glaze Icing

- Juice of 1/4 Lemon
- 3 Tbsp. Powdered Erythritol

Directions

1. Mix the dry ingredients together. Add the egg and combine until you achieve the sticky dough.

2. Bring oil to 375F. Drop 4 dough balls at a time. Brown on one side and flip over – total 4 minutes.

3. Remove from the pan.

4. In a small bowl, combine the erythritol and lemon juice until icing is set.

5. Serve and enjoy!

Each serving contains 50 calories, 4.5g fat, 0.7g carbs, and 1.7g protein.

DESSERT RECIPES

KETO LEMON BERRY POPSICLES

Ingredients

- 100g Raspberries
- 1 cup Coconut Milk
- Juice 1/2 Lemon
- 20 drops Liquid Stevia
- 1/4 cup Sour Cream
- 1/4 cup Heavy Cream
- 1/4 cup Coconut Oil
- 1/2 tsp. Guar Gum

Directions

1. Add the ingredients together in a container. Use a blender to combine the mixture together.

2. Strain the mixture and pour into the molds. Freeze for 2 hours.

3. Serve immediately and enjoy!

Each serving contains 150 calories, 16g fat, 2g carbs, and 0.6g protein.

NEAPOLITAN BARS

Ingredients

- ¼ cup Butter
- ¼ cup Coconut Oil
- ¼ cup Cream Cheese
- ¼ cup Sour Cream
- 1 tbsp. Cocoa Powder
- 1 tbsp. Erythritol
- 14 drops Liquid Steve
- ½ tsp. Vanilla extract,
- 2 strawberries

Directions

1. Except the vanilla, strawberries, cocoa powder, combine the ingredients in a blender and mix until well combined.

2. Separate into 3 bowls and add cocoa to one, strawberries to another and vanilla to the last. Pour the chocolate mixture into a mold then freeze for 30 minutes. Pour the strawberry and vanilla layers and repeat.

3. Freeze for at least 1 hour.

4. Serve and enjoy!

Each serving contains 51 calories, 5.4g fat, 0.2g carbs, and 0.3g protein.

NO-BAKE PEANUT BUTTER CHOCOLATE BALLS

Ingredients

- 1/4 cup Coconut oil
- 3 tbsp. Cocoa Powder
- 2 tbsp. PB fit powder
- 3 tbsp. Shelled Hemp Seeds
- ½ tsp. Vanilla extract
- 14 drops liquid Stevia
- ¼ Unsweetened Shredded Coconut

Directions

1. Mix the dry ingredients together with the coconut oil. Add vanilla, heavy cream, and liquid stevia. Mix until well combined.

2. Place the shredded coconut onto a plate. Roll the mixture into balls roll in the unsweetened shredded coconut.

3. Add the balls onto a baking tray lined in parchment paper and place in the freezer for about 20 minutes.

4. Serve and enjoy!

Each serving contains 104 calories, 10g fat, 0.4g carbs, and 2.2g protein.

KETO TROPICAL SMOOTHIE

Ingredients

- 3/4 cup Unsweetened Coconut Milk
- 1/4 cup Sour Cream
- 2 tbsp. Golden Flaxseed Meal
- 1 tbsp. Olive Oil
- 1/2 tsp. Mango Extract
- 1/4 tsp. Banana Extract
- 1/4 tsp. Blueberry Extract
- 20 drops Liquid Stevia
- 6 Ice Cubes

Directions

1. Add all the ingredients together into a blender. Let the mixture sit for at least 3 minutes for the flax meal to soak. Blend until well combined.

2. Serve immediately and enjoy!

Each serving contains 351 calories, 30.8g fat, 3g carbs, and 4.9g protein.

SPINACH CUCUMBER SMOOTHIE

Ingredients

- 1 Cucumber, peeled and cubed
- 2 handfuls Spinach
- 1 cup Coconut Milk
- 1 tbsp. Olive Oil
- 1/4 tsp. Xanthan Gum
- 12 drops Liquid Stevia
- 7 Ice Cubes

Directions

1. Add all the ingredients together into a blender. Blend until well combined.

2. Serve immediately and enjoy!

Each serving contains 334 calories, 33g fat, 3g carbs, and 4g protein.

KETO CHOCOLATE MACAROONS

Ingredients

- 20 grams Sugar-free Chocolate
- 1 Egg white
- 1 cup Shredded Coconut
- 1/4 cup Erythritol
- 2 tbsp. Coconut Oil
- 1/2 tsp. Almond Extract
- 1 pinch of Salt

Directions

1. Preheat oven to 350 F.

2. Spread the coconut into a thin layer on a lined baking sheet. Bake for 5 minutes, until toasted.

3. Beat the egg white until foamy. Then add salt, erythritol, and almond extract slowly while mixing. Once the coconut is toasted, combine with the mixture.

4. Using a small scoop, tightly spoon balls of macaroon batter and place them on parchment paper. Bake until golden - 15 minutes.

5. While baking, make the chocolate drizzle by melting sugar-free chocolate and coconut oil, stirring frequently. Once the macaroons are baked, drizzle chocolate over them.

6. Serve and enjoy!

Each serving contains 73.2 calories, 7.3g fat, 2.7g carbs, and 1g protein.

KETO CHOCOLATE PEANUT BUTTER TARTS

Ingredients

Crust

- 1/4 cup Flaxseeds
- 2 tbsp. Almond Flour
- 1 tbsp. Erythritol
- 1 Egg White

Top Layer

- 1 Avocado
- 4 tbsps. Cocoa Powder
- 2 tbsp. Heavy Cream
- 1/4 cup Erythritol
- 1/2 tsp. Cinnamon
- 1/2 tsp. Vanilla Extract

Middle Layer

- 4 tbsps. Peanut Butter
- 2 tbsps. Butter

Directions

1. Preheat your oven to 350 F.

2. Grind the flaxseeds and combine with the crust ingredients. Press the mixture into tart pans and bake for 8 minutes or until set.

3. Combine the top layer ingredients and blender until smooth. Allow the crust to cool. Melt the butter and peanut butter in the microwave and pour onto your tart crusts. Let chill for 30 minutes until set. Add the avocado chocolate layer on top and even out. Let chill for another 30 minutes.

4. Serve and enjoy!

Each serving contains 304.8 calories, 26.8g fat, 10.5g carbs, and 9.8g protein.

PECAN PUMPKIN ICE CREAM

Ingredients

- 3 Egg Yolks
- 2 cups Coconut Milk
- 1/2 cup Pumpkin Puree
- 1/2 cup Cottage Cheese
- 1/2 cup Pecans, toasted
- 1/3 cup Erythritol
- 2 tbsp. Butter, salted
- 1 tsp. Maple Extract
- 1 tsp. Pumpkin Spice
- 1/2 tsp. Xanthan Gum
- 20 drops Liquid Stevia

Directions

1. Chop the toasted pecans and pour into the stove with butter. Place the ingredients in a blender and mix.
2. Add the mixture to your ice cream machine and add the butter and pecans. Follow the instructions of your ice cream maker.
3. Serve and enjoy!

Each serving contains 248.3 calories, 22.3g fat, 7.1g carbs, and 6.5g protein.

KETO PUMPKIN BLONDIES

Ingredients

- 1 Egg
- 1 oz. Pecans, chopped
- 1/2 cup Pumpkin Puree
- 1/2 cup Butter- softened
- 1/2 cup Erythritol
- 1/4 cup Almond Flour
- 2 tbsp. Coconut Flour
- 1 tsp. Maple Extract
- 1 tsp. Cinnamon
- 1/8 tsp. Pumpkin Pie Spice
- 15 drops Liquid Stevia

Directions

1. Preheat your oven to 350F.

2. Add the egg, softened butter, erythritol, and pumpkin puree into the mixer. Stir I coconut flour, almond flour, stevia, cinnamon, maple extract, and pumpkin pie spice.

3. Spray a pan with coconut oil and pour the batter. Sprinkle pecans over the top and bake for 20 minutes until top is set and golden.

4. Serve and enjoy!

Each serving contains 111.5 calories, 10.8g fat, 2.8g carbs, and 1.4g protein.

KETO SNICKER DOODLE PUMPKIN COOKIES

Ingredients

Cookies

- 1 large Egg
- 1 1/2 cups Almond Flour
- 1/2 cup Pumpkin Puree
- 1/4 cup Butter, salted
- 1/4 cup Erythritol
- 1 tsp. Vanilla Extract
- 1/2 tsp. Baking Powder
- 25 drops Liquid Stevia

Topping

- 2 tsp. Erythritol
- 1 tsp. Pumpkin Pie Spice

Directions

1. Preheat oven to 350 F.

2. Combine the dry ingredients and mix. In a separate bowl, measure the vanilla, liquid stevia, pumpkin puree, and butter. Mix until well combined and dough is formed. Roll the dough into balls and place on a lined cookie sheet.

3. Flatten the balls with your hands and bake for 12 minutes.

4. Combine pumpkin pie spice and erythritol in a grinder. Once the cookies are baked, sprinkle and top and let cool.

Each serving contains 98.7calories, 8.9g fat, 3.2g carbs, and 2.9g protein.

KETO NO-BAKE PUMPKIN CHEESECAKE

Ingredients

The Crust

- 25 drops Liquid Stevia
- 1/2 cup Flaxseed Meal
- 3/4 cup Almond Flour
- 1/4 cup Butter
- 1 tsp. Pumpkin Pie Spice

The Filling

- 25 drops Liquid Stevia
- 4 oz. Cream Cheese
- 1/3 cup Pumpkin Puree
- 1/4 cup Heavy Cream
- 3 tbsp. Butter
- 2 tbsp. Sour Cream
- 1/4 tsp. Pumpkin Pie Spice

Directions

1. Combine the dry ingredients for the crust then add the stevia and butter. Form small balls of a dough and press into the pans.

2. Combine the filling ingredients and blend until smooth. Pour the mixture into the crusts and chill for 4 hours.

3. Serve and enjoy!

Each serving contains 264.5 calories, 25.3g fat, 6.5g carbs, and 5g protein.

KETO PEANUT BUTTER FUDGE

Ingredients

Crust

- 1/4 cup Butter, melted
- 1 cup Almond Flour
- 1/2 tsp. Cinnamon
- 1 tbsp. Erythritol
- Salt

Fudge

- 1/2 cup Peanut Butter
- 1/4 cup Heavy cream
- 1/4 cup Butter, melted
- 1/4 cup Erythritol
- 1/2 tsp. Vanilla Extract
- 1/8 tsp. Xanthan Gum

Toppings

- 1/3 cup Chocolate, chopped

Directions

1. Preheat oven to 400 F. Combine melted butter, erythritol, almond flour, salt, and cinnamon. Mix until well combined then press into the baking dish.

2. Bake for 10 minutes. And let cool.

3. Combine the fudge ingredients in a blender then spread the fudge evenly over the dish. Top with chopped chocolate and let chill overnight.

Each serving contains 299.5 calories, 19.75g fat, 8.75g carbs, and 4g protein.

KETO STRAWBERRY ICE CREAM

Ingredients

3 Egg Yolks

1 cup Heavy Cream

1/3 cup Erythritol

1/2 tsp. Vanilla Extract

1/8 tsp. Xanthan Gum

1 cup Strawberries, pureed

Directions

1. Pour heavy cream into a pot over low heat. Add the erythritol and let dissolve.

2. Separate 3 egg whites in a mixing bowl and mix until doubled in size. Slowly add in the hot cream mixture while continuing the beat the eggs. Add the vanilla extract and mix.

3. Allow the mixture to freeze for 2 hours or use an ice cream mixture.

4. Once the ice cream has thickened, add the strawberry puree. Mix into the ice cream but don't over mix. Allow the ice cream to chill overnight.

5. Serve and enjoy!

Each serving contains 178 calories, 16.9g fat, 3.3g carbs, and 2.3g protein.

KETO STRAWBERRY SHORTCAKES

Ingredients

Keto Puff Cakes

- 3 Eggs
- 3 oz. Cream Cheese
- 2 tbsp. Erythritol
- 1/2 tsp. Vanilla
- 1/4 tsp. Baking Powder

Filling

- 10 Strawberries
- 1 cup Heavy Cream

Directions

1. Preheat oven to 300 F.

2. Beat the egg whites until fluffy.

3. In a container, add cream cheese, baking powder, vanilla, erythritol and eggs. Mix until smooth.

4. Fold the egg whites into the egg yolk mixture and evenly spread on a baking sheet.

5. Bake for 25 minutes. Top with strawberries and whipped cream.

6. Serve and enjoy!

Each serving contains 270 calories, 28.2g fat, 3.9g carbs, and 5g protein.

BROWN BUTTER PECAN ICE CREAM

Ingredients

- 1 1/2 cups Unsweetened Coconut Milk
- 1/4 cup Pecans, crushed
- 1/4 cup Heavy Cream
- 5 tbsp. Butter
- 1/4 tsp. Xanthan Gum
- 25 drops Liquid Stevia

Directions

1. Brown the butter over low heat. Stir in the stevia, cream, and pecans and mix well.

2. Whisk the xanthan gum and coconut milk into the brown butter mix then stir into the ice cream machine.

3. Follow according to the ice cream maker.

4. Serve and enjoy!

Each serving contains 318.7 calories, 35.3g fat, 3.3g carbs, and 0.7g protein.

SEA SALT BUTTERSCOTCH ICE CREAM

Ingredients

- 1 cup Coconut Milk
- 1/4 cup Heavy Cream
- 1/4 cup Sour Cream
- 3 tbsp. Butter, browned
- 2 tbsp. Erythritol
- 2 tsp. Butterscotch Flavoring
- 1 tsp. Flaked Sea Salt
- 1/2 tsp. Xanthan Gum
- 25 drops Liquid Stevia

Directions

1. Brown the butter. Add all ingredients to a blender and mix.

2. Pour into the ice cream maker and follow directions accordingly.

3. Serve and enjoy!

Each serving contains 245.3 calories, 24.0g fat, 2.3g carbs, and 0.7g protein.

KETO MOCHA ICE CREAM

Ingredients

- 1 cup Coconut Milk
- 1/4 cup Heavy Cream
- 2 tbsp. Cocoa Powder
- 2 tbsp. Erythritol
- 1 tbsp. Instant Coffee
- 1/4 tsp. Xanthan Gum
- 15 drops Liquid Stevia

Directions

1. Excerpt the xanthan gum, add all ingredients into a container and blend with an immersion blender.

2. Slowly add the xanthan gum until a thick mixture is formed. Pour into your ice cream maker and follow directions accordingly.

3. Serve immediately and enjoy!

Each serving contains 145 calories, 15g fat, 4g carbs, and 1g protein.

KETO HOT COCOA

Ingredients

- 1 1/2 Cup Unsweetened Coconut Milk
- 2 Tbsp. Unsweetened Cocoa Powder
- 2 Tbsp. Heavy Cream
- 1 Tbsp. Splenda
- 1 tsp. Instant Coffee
- 1/2 tsp. Cinnamon
- 1/2 tsp. Vanilla Extract

Directions

1. Pour coconut milk and heavy cream in a saucepan over medium heat.

2. Allow the milk mixture to steam. Add your coffee and cinnamon. Mix well.

3. Add cocoa powder, vanilla and Splenda. Stir until well-combined.

4. Increase the heat to high heat, coming into a boil.

5. Once the mixture is boiling, reduce to low heat continue to stir.

6. Serve immediately and enjoy!

Each serving contains 206 calories, 18g fat, 13g carbs, and 2g protein.

CHOCOLATE CHERRY DONUTS

Ingredients

- 2 large Eggs
- 5 10g bars Dark Choco Perfection
- 3/4 cup Almond Flour
- 1/4 cup Golden Flaxseed Meal
- 3 tbsp. Coconut Milk (from the carton)
- 3 tbsp. Sweet Perfection
- 2 1/2 tbsp. Coconut Oil
- 1 tsp. Baking Powder
- 1 tsp. Vanilla Extract
- 2 tsp. Berry Extract of Choice
- Pinch Salt

Directions

1. Mix all wet ingredients into the batter. Chop the chocolate bars into chunks and fold into the batter. Add the berry extract.

2. Heat your donut maker and lightly grease. Pour the batter and cook for 4-5 minutes each. Flip each donut and cook for another 2 minutes.

3. Repeat until mixture is complete. Set aside.

4. Serve immediately and enjoy!

Each serving contains 106.7 calories, 9.4g fat, 6.8g carbs, and 3.1g protein.

CONDIMENTS

KETO RASPBERRY VINAIGRETTE

Ingredients

- 1/2 cup Golden Raspberries
- 1/2 cup Extra Virgin Olive Oil
- 1/2 cup White Wine Vinegar
- 25 drops Stevia

Directions

1. Combine all ingredients in a blender and mix until well combined.

2. Strain the seeds out and set the liquids aside. Use on all of your favorite salads. Enjoy!

Each serving contains 85 Calories, 9.3g Fats, 0.3g Net Carbs, and 1g Protein.

KETO PESTO SAUCE

Ingredients

- 1.5 cups Basil
- 1/3 cup Pine Nuts
- 2/3 cup Olive Oil
- 3/4 cup Parmesan Cheese
- 2 tsps. Tomato Paste
- 1 tsp. Minced Garlic
- Salt and Pepper, to taste

Directions

1. Except the oil, add the entire remaining ingredient to a jar.

2. Using an immersion blender, mix the ingredients together. Slowly stir in the olive oil.

3. Store in a sealed jar.

Each serving contains 84 Calories, 8.9g Fats, 0.4g Net Carbs, and 1.3g Protein

GUACAMOLE

Ingredients

- 2 medium avocados
- 3 cup cherry tomatoes
- 1 white onion
- 1 lime – juiced
- 4 tbsp. freshly chopped cilantro
- 4 cloves garlic
- Salt and pepper

Directions

1. Combine all ingredients into the bowl and mash until well-combined. Chill for 10 minutes.

2. Serve immediately and enjoy!

Each serving contains 180 calories, 15g fat, 13g carbs, and 2.7g protein.

KETO MAPLE SYRUP

Ingredients

- 3/4 Cup Water
- 1/4 Cup Erythritol
- 1 Tbsp. Butter
- 2 ½ tsps. Coconut Oil
- 2 tsps. Maple Extract
- 1/2 tsp. Vanilla Extract
- 1/4 tsp. Xanthan Gum

Directions

1. In a bowl, mix coconut oil, butter, and xanthan gum together. Microwave for 45 seconds.

2. Grind the erythritol until fine powdered results.

3. Combine the water, oils, and erythritol Add the maple extract, vanilla extract, and stevia for desired taste.

4. Microwave for 60 seconds, stirring frequently.

5. Serve and enjoy!

Each serving contains 49 Calories, 5.5g Fats, 0g Net Carbs, and 0g Protein.

KETO MAYONNAISE

Ingredients

- 1 cup olive oil
- 1 egg, room temp
- 2 egg yolks, room temp
- 1 Tbsp. whey
- 1 tsp. Dijon mustard
- 1 tsp. salt
- 1 tsp. smoked paprika
- 3 stevia drops liquid

Directions

1. Add all ingredients except olive oil in your blender. Slowly begin blending as you add one drop of oil at a time.

2. As the mayonnaise starts to emulsify, add more oil until full.

3. Store in a jar with lid and refrigerate.

Each serving contains 137 Calories, 14.6 Fats, 0g Net Carbs, and 0.6g Protein.

CONCLUSION

As we reach the end of this book and you've learned all there is to know about the ketogenic diet, allow me to welcome you to the world of optimum health!

The studies that have been done on the ketogenic diet have been proven to be safe and actually work better than most traditional diets. Whether you are trying to lose weight, improve a chronic disease that will respond to metabolic chances or simply trying to live a healthier lifestyle, the ketogenic lifestyle will make your life so much easier.

I hope that you will find the information in the book to be helpful and intriguing enough to inspire you to learn more about this particular diet and try it. Through extensive knowledge, experience and preparation, it is hoped that this eBook is all you need to get started on your journey to better health. As the internet is full of informative websites that will provide more information than a thousand books, always be sure that you use information from a credible source.

While this doesn't mean that you should not follow the recipes from someone's ketogenic-themed blog, you must be sure that they are accurately following the diet before trusting their recipes and information. The worst thing you can do is to use recipes that end up sabotaging your diet by getting too little protein or too many carbohydrates.

Finally, make sure to stick to the plan! The Ketogenic diet plan is a wonderful improvement to your body. Unfortunately, cheating on a regular basis will actually set back your dietary success. As mentioned earlier, you shouldn't beat yourself up when it comes to counting macros , but that doesn't mean that you can have a delicious deep dish pizza or a fully loaded baked potato either. With some will power and motivation, you will find that choosing the Keto diet is actually quite easy to follow.

Remember that the Keto diet gives you the freedom to change the kinds of foods you eat and satisfy your hunger. Experiment with the recipes you find here and see if you can enhance that in any way to make them better. The ketogenic diet isn't just about eating great – it's about eating right!

www.ingramcontent.com/pod-product-compliance
Lightning Source LLC
Chambersburg PA
CBHW051957280526
45793CB00005B/760